AF616773

THERAPEUTIC EXERCISE

F.H. Ewerhardt
Gertrude F. Riddle

SHREE PUBLISHERS & DISTRIBUTORS
NEW DELHI-110 002

Edition : 2011

Published by :
SHREE PUBLISHERS & DISTRIBUTORS
22/4735 Prakash Deep Building,
Ansari Road, Darya Ganj,
New Delhi–110 002

ISBN : 978–81–89329–467–6

Printed by :
Vikas Computers & Printers
Naveen Shahdara, Delhi–110 032

PREFACE

It is the intention of the authors of this manual to provide students training in physical education, occupational therapy, and physical therapy with a manual which will be concise in content and yet will not contain too much irrelevant material. The subject matter is, to a large extent, material which both authors have been using in their class work; one at Washington University School of Medicine and the other at St. Louis University.

Students interested in the proper application of therapeutic exercise should be particularly well informed regarding the musculature of the extremities, shoulder and hip girdles. For this reason in this volume only enough anatomy is included to satisfy the immediate requirements. The student will refer to the more comprehensive texts in anatomy for references whenever the need should arise.

The art of applying therapeutic exercise is necessarily closely related to kinesiology, which is the science of bodily movements. Therefore, considerable space is devoted to the classification and general characteristics of muscular action. Members of the medical profession, with few exceptions, regard passive, resistive, and active voluntary exercises as about the same thing; namely, just exercise. It is hoped that this volume, in addition to its prime objective, may do its part in educating the general practitioner, and particularly the orthopedic surgeon, to an appreciation of the differential value of these various forms of movements.

F. H. E.
G. F. R.

St. Louis, Missouri

CONTENTS

CHAPTER I

Introduction to Therapeutic Exercise

CHAPTER II

Analysis of Joint Motion

CHAPTER III

Brief Review of Muscles Participating in Joint Movements

CHAPTER IV

Physiology of Skeletal Muscle

CHAPTER V

Plexuses of Nerves Controlling the Upper and Lower Extremities

CHAPTER VI

Physiology of Therapeutic Exercise

CHAPTER VII

Special Applications of Therapeutic Exercise

CHAPTER VIII

Application of Therapeutic Exercise in Medicine

CHAPTER IX

POLIOMYELITIS

CHAPTER X

SPASTIC PARALYSIS

THERAPEUTIC EXERCISE

CHAPTER I

INTRODUCTION TO THERAPEUTIC EXERCISE

Brief History of Therapeutic Exercise.—Physical activity has been related to the practice of medicine almost since the beginning of recorded history. According to the account of a Chinese priest, a series of medical exercises called Cong Fu were known and practiced in China as early as 2600 B. C. More comprehensively chronicled are the physical exercises which played a part in the lives of the Greeks and of the Romans. The physical training embraced a wide variety of activities directed toward encouraging the complete development of the individual, both for esthetic and for military reasons.

In the 18th century, Gutsmann and Froebel of Germany developed systems whose aims were the strengthening and harmonizing of body and soul. It was also in this period that Ludwig Jahn originated the Turnverein. His objectives were mainly patriotic—to develop youth physically in order to equip the nation for defense. In Sweden, Spiess and Henrik Ling founded the Swedish system, still widely practiced throughout the world. Swedish gymnastics, unlike Jahn's Turnverein system, are designed for the individual rather than for the group. Physical perfection is the aim, each series of movements being based strictly on physiological laws. England's contribution is mainly in the field of sports, the chief objective being recreation and fitness.

In the United States since 1855 there has been an increasing interest in physical education with the introduction of numerous systems under various names and attempts have been made to combine odds and ends of several to form a unified whole. In general, the trend today is toward national sport activities, less formal gymnastics and the introduction of corrective gymnastics in the public school systems.

Principles of Therapeutic Exercise.—In recent years there has developed an awareness of the importance of efficiency in order to maintain healthful living. Increasing emphasis has been placed on reaching a balance between work and play, mental and physical effort. The value of physical efficiency lies particularly in the fact that an individual can perform his work more easily, that he has a better endurance, that he can recover from a given task more rapidly and that he can enjoy the actual doing more, if he has equipped himself by the intelligent use of exercise.

The true value of exercise is not to be found in the theory that increased muscle bulk is synonymous with good health or the accomplishment of specialized athletic feats. On the contrary, the benefits of exercise are to be found in the attainment of physical poise, the ability to perform work with the least expenditure of energy and the furtherance of proper activity of tissue and organs. Muscle re-education aims to re-establish neuromuscular pathways by the practice of coördinated movements of balance, skill, and those requiring a discriminative appreciation of spatial relationship of one part of the body to another. This performance demands precise, conscious, thoughtfully directed effort which may be aroused only by discerning, purposeful, voluntary exercise and cannot be brought about by passive movements.

General Characteristics of Muscular Action.—In the selection of appropriate exercises it is important to recognize certain principles relating to muscular action.

It is generally believed that the voluntary contraction of one muscle or set of muscles influences the relaxation of the opposing muscle or group of muscles. This principle is applied when resistive exercise is employed to reduce spasms and lessen the action of the antagonistic group of muscles.

A second important principle is that each muscle may be regarded as possessing a special function.

A third is the recognition that with any muscular action numerous muscle synergists supplement the action of the prime mover.

The following generalizations may prove helpful in planning a régime of muscle training.

A muscle group in need of strengthening should not be called upon to perform its maximum load at the beginning of training. It is more desirable to exercise often in small doses than a few times in large doses. The capacity for work is greater if at no time the muscle is pushed to its limit; exercise may be carried to the point of fatigue, but not beyond this point. This is especially true in the treatment of paralyses.

The greater the frequency of contraction, the more rapid the approach of fatigue; the more complete the exhaustion, mental or muscular, the longer the period necessary for recovery. The more complex the discriminations required in a performance, the more rapid the onset of fatigue. A patient suffering from nervous exhaustion, for example, should not be asked to play a game unfamiliar to him.

Definitions.—*Therapeutic Exercise or Corrective Exercise.*—Therapeutic exercise may be defined as the specialized application of bodily movements scientifically designed to maintain or to restore normal muscle, nerve, and joint function.

Kinesiology.—Kinesiology is the scientific study of human motion.

Muscle Re-education.—Muscle re-education is that form of therapeutic exercise given to muscles in which principally the neuro-muscular coördination has in some way become disturbed, disrupted, or even partially destroyed.

CHAPTER II

ANALYSIS OF JOINT MOTION

CLASSIFICATION OF ARTICULATIONS ANATOMICALLY

Types of Articulation.

1. Diarthrosis—is a freely movable joint, or the true joint, in which there is a joint cavity, articular capsule, synovial membrane and fluid.
2. Synarthrosis—is a fixed joint in which no movement is possible.
3. Amphiarthrosis—is a slightly movable joint.

Description of Articulations.

1. Diarthrodial Articulation and Movements.
   - (*a*) A Spheroidal joint is composed of a rounded head in a concave surface, as the metacarpophalangeal joints.
   - (*b*) An Enarthrosis, or ball and socket joint, is composed of a head locked in a socket which is more than a hemisphere, as the femur.
   - (*c*) A Hinge or ginglymus joint displays movement on a plane at right angle to the axis, as the interphalangeal joints.
   - (*d*) A Screw joint is a hinge joint in which movement is not at right angle to the axis, as the atlanto-epistropheal joint.
   - (*e*) Ellipsodial joint is one in which a convex surface is received in a concave surface, as the radiocarpal articulation.
   - (*f*) Trochoidal, or pivot, joint is one in which the edge of a disk glides in a corresponding groove, as the superior and inferior radio-ulnar articulations.
   - (*g*) A Saddle joint is one in which the bone is concave in one direction and convex in another, and the bony articulation with it is the opposite to fit into it, as the metacarpophalangeal joint of the thumb.
   - (*h*) The Arthrodial, or gliding, joints are the vertebral articulations.

Movements of the Diarthrodial Joint.

(*a*) Gliding or slipping as in the radio-ulnar joints.

(*b*) Rolling—there is no pure rolling but combined with gliding gives,
(*c*) Mixed gliding and rolling as in the femoral condyle, which involves rolling and at the same time slipping upon the superior articulating surface of the tibia.
(*d*) Rotation is ideal not real, and is the gliding of one curved surface upon a fixed curved surface resulting in the turning of a segment of a body on its long axis.
(*e*) Mixed gliding, rolling and rotation occurs at the knee when it is at the completion of extension.

2. Synarthrodial Articulations.
(*a*) Synchrondrosis (connected by cartilage).
(*b*) Suture:
Serrate, saw toothed.
Squamous, beveled edges of two bones overlap.
Hormonic, regular edges united by fibrous tissue.
Gomphosis is the union of the roots of teeth with the walls of the dental alveoli.
(*c*) Syndesmosis (connected by ligaments).
(*a*) Cord form—as the stylohyoid ligament.
(*b*) Band form—as the coracoacromial ligament.
(*d*) Synostosis is an irregular form of union of bone by osseous matter which occurs more normally in many synchrondrosis or suture types, never in the syndesmosis type.

3. Amphiarthrodial Articulation (slightly movable). This is a term connoting structure in which there is a progesssive development in the joint toward diarthrosis but in which the movement is slight. The commonly accepted meaning is that of employing restricted motion as in the symphysis pubis and vertebræ.

NORMAL JOINT MOVEMENTS

Glossary of Joint Motion Definitions.

Retraction:	Movement backward, as of the shoulder.
Protraction:	Movement forward, as of the shoulder.
Abduction:	Movement away from midline.
Adduction:	Movement toward midline.
Flexion:	Is to bend a segment at the joint, or to decrease the joint angle.
Extension:	Is to straighten a segment at the joint, or to increase the joint angle.

External or Lateral Rotation:	Is to revolve on an axis away from midline.
Internal or Medial Rotation:	Is to revolve on an axis toward midline.
Circumduction:	Is a combination of all movements or a motion in which the distal end of a segment describes a circle and the proximal end the sides of a cone.
Supination:	Is to turn the anterior side upward.
Pronation:	Is to turn the anterior side downward.
Inversion:	Is the same as supination.
Eversion:	Is the same as pronation.

A. Shoulder Movements:

1. Abduction
2. Adduction
3. Flexion
4. Extension
5. Rotation—lateral
6. Rotation—medial
7. Protraction
8. Retraction
9. Circumduction

B. Elbow Movements:

1. Flexion
2. Extension
3. Supination
4. Pronation

C. Wrist Movements:

1. Flexion
2. Extension
3. Ulnar abduction
4. Radial abduction
5. Circumduction

D. Hip Movements:

1. Flexion
2. Extension
3. Abduction
4. Adduction
5. Internal rotation
6. External rotation
7. Circumduction

E. Knee Movements:

1. Flexion
2. Extension
3. With knee flexed some rotation

F. Ankle Movements:

1. Flexion (dorsi-flexion)
2. Extension (plantar-flexion)
3. Inversion (supination)
4. Eversion (pronation)
5. Circumduction

Factors Influencing Normal Range of Motion.—Because of the influence of gravity, the relation of other muscles to the skeleton. and positional factors, a given muscle may perform functions which would not be deduced from a simple study of the relation of the muscle to the skeleton. For instance, through the action of gravity the psoas iliacus not only flexes the hip, but also apparently is concerned with flexing the knee; and the hamstring muscles while extending the hip seem to extend the knee.

Determination of Planes of Movement.—The axes about which a bone moves at a given joint are frequently complex—therefore, for practical purposes, it is usually possible to determine an approximate axis about which any given movement takes place.

From this standpoint diarthrodial joints may be divided into three groups:

1. *Uniaxial Joints.*—In the uniaxial joints movements of note may be made merely about one approximate axis. If a muscle acts on such a joint, it exerts an effective pull either in one direction about this axis or in the opposite direction. Most joints of this sort are of the hinge type, capable of flexion and extension. In joints of the pivot type (as the joint between the dens and the atlas) the movement is one of rotation.

2. *Biaxial Joints.*—In the biaxial joints there are two approximated primary axes of movement. Muscles acting on such a joint may cause movement about either axis—or intermediate axis. Examples are the metacarpal joint of the thumb and the wrist joint; about one axis flexion and extension occur; about the other axis, abduction and adduction. A given muscle may cause movement about one axis or both axes.

3. *Multiaxial Joints.*—In multiaxial joints movements may be made about the axis in three directions, each plane vertical to each of the other planes. Joints of this type are called ball and socket (enarthrosis).

The muscles controlling joint movements are prime movers aided or controlled by other groups called synergists. Those muscles opposing the movement (or producing movement in an opposite direction) are called antagonists.

If all joints were of the uniaxial type, it would be relatively easy to arrange the muscles acting on joints into synergists and antagonists, although even in such joints a muscle might be so attached that it would be a "flexor" after flexion has started, an "extensor" after extension has started. In case of biaxial, and still more so in case of multiaxial joints, the direction of pull exerted by a given muscle with respect to a given axis varies so much with the position of the articulating bones that muscles which in one position are antagonists in another position become synergists during the same general movement.

Terms of Position and Direction.—All definitions are on the supposition that the body is in an upright position with arms at the sides and palms facing forward, the anatomical position.

1. Ventral or anterior is to the front of the body.
2. Dorsal or posterior is to the rear of the body.
3. Cranial or superior is toward the head.
4. Caudal or inferior is toward the feet.
5. The mid-sagittal plane is the medial line of the body.
6. Lateral is away from the midline plane.
7. Internal is deeper, nearer the central axis of the body or a part.
8. External is superficial in position.
9. Proximal is near the trunk.
10. Distal is peripheral.

There are three fundamental planes of the body in which motion may take place:

1. Sagittal plane is a vertical plane through the longitudinal axis of the trunk. Dividing the body into right and left halves is the mid-sagittal plane, and any plane parallel to it is a sagittal plane.

2. A transverse, or horizontal, plane is a plane across the body at a right angle to sagittal or coronal planes.

3. A frontal, or coronal, plane is any vertical plane at a right angle to a sagittal plane and dividing the body into anterior and posterior positions.

LEVERS

Description of Levers of the Body.—Movement in any machine is brought about by a force acting on a lever. In the human body the bones act as the levers, the muscles supply the power which produces the movement, and the joints themselves act as the fulcra. Principles of mechanical action, as governing machines, may be applied to the human body; however, the mechanical action of muscles is far more complex. A knowledge of basic mechanical action of bones, joints, and muscles responsible for bodily functions is necessary for an understanding of therapeutic exercise. It is only by the action of muscles on these bony levers that man can stand erect, have locomotion, and impart movement to other objects.

There are three orders of levers encountered in the human skeletal system:

1. In levers of the first order the fulcrum (joint) lies between the weight (resistance to be overcome) and the power (which is applied by the muscle at its point of insertion).

2. In levers of the second order the weight (resistance to be overcome) lies between the point of application of power (insertion of a muscle) and the fulcrum (joint).

3. Levers of the third order—this is the commonest type found in the body. The power (insertion of the muscle) lies between the weight (resistance to be overcome) and the fulcrum (joint).

Examples of Levers of the Body.

1. *Examples of the First Order of Levers.*—The sternocleidomastoid, acting singly, bends the head obliquely downwards toward the shoulder of the same side. This muscle then, when it acts singly, does not rotate the head, so as to carry the face toward the opposite side. Its fulcrum or center of motion is the articulation between the occiput and the upper surface of the atlas. Rotation does not take place at this articulation. The movement is flexion and extension at the articulation between the occiput and the atlas, and represents a striking example of the first order of leverage. In the backward movement of the head, the dorsal or extension muscles represent the power; the front of the head represents the weight to be raised; and between the power and weight is the fulcrum, or center of motion, at the occipito-atlantal articulation. Also of the first order is the foot flexed or extended with the patient in the sitting position. A cross section of the trunk at any given level shows that the axis is the intervertebral articulation, the force is either abdominal flexors or back extensors, and the resistance (weight) is the respective antagonist or weight of the trunk.

2. *Examples of the Second Order of Levers.*—In levers of the second order, the point on which the power is exerted moves through a greater distance than the point of resistance. Speed of motion is thus sacrificed to power.

(*a*) The position of standing on the toes illustrates the fulcrum (the contact between the toe joint and the floor) with the weight or resistance that part of the body which is applied to the astragalus. The power is the insertion of the gastrocnemius muscle tendon on the calcaneus.

(*b*) The triceps may be considered a lever of the second order if the movement is made from a flexed position of the forearm. The weight is then between the fulcrum and the power. Insertion of the triceps muscle is on the olecranon process of the ulna and the humero-ulnar joint.

3. *Examples of the Third Order of Levers.*—In levers of the third class, the point on which the force is exerted moves through less distance than the point of resistance. Power is thus sacrificed

to speed. This is the commonest form of leverage found in the body.

(*a*) The bending of the elbow to lift a weight resting on the hand presents the elbow joint as the fulcrum, the insertion of the brachialis muscle (coronoid process of the ulna) as the power, and the object in the hand as the weight.

(*b*) Besides the example given above, most of the hip and knee muscles operate those segments as levers of the third class. In this type lever a movement of the point of power through a short distance will cause (weight or resistance to be overcome) to move through a greater distance.

Levers and Their Mechanical Relationship to Muscles.—The more the angle between a muscle or its tendon and the bone on which it acts approaches a right angle, the greater is the power of movement exerted by the muscle. All boys know it is easier to "chin" oneself when the arm is partly bent than when hanging straight from a bar. Therefore, since most of the muscles run nearly parallel with the parts on which they act, the tendons, before their attachments, are usually carried over either a bony prominence or some fascia or ligament, thus making it act as a pulley and causing the tendon to act as if it were inserted at an oblique angle. At other times, a process for the attachment of a tendon projects from the bone and causes the force of the contracting muscle to be more advantageously exerted on the bone. It may be seen readily that the greater the distance of the attachment of a muscle from the joint on which it acts, the greater will be the power of a muscle. Conversely, the more nearly parallel the termination of a muscle is to the axis of the bone into which it is inserted, the weaker will be its action.

The mechanical action of bones, joints, and muscles is of extreme importance to a régime of re-education, as the normal functioning of this mechanism is essential to good health. It is significant that regardless of whether the various levers are of the first, second, or third order they are usually so arranged that the distance between the fulcrum and point of application of power is short. The body is adapted primarily to the production of rapid movements against slight resistance. Also, it should be noted that in the presence of slight pathological contraction of muscles, there may be a relatively marked angulation of a joint. It is also true that a muscle which has become weakened for any reason may be working at a disadvantage because of its short leverage.

These points are of clinical importance to an understanding of the physiological shortening resulting when a muscle develops spasm on account of nature's protective mechanism set in motion at the time of injury to the bone or joint. Failure to relax the spastic group, after the need for protection has passed, results in a physiological shortening of the muscle group, and forms an ideal setting for the development of contractures and adhesions.

The mechanical action of muscles and joints plays an extremely important rôle in the aftermath of stiffened joints with formation of adhesions and resultant limitation of motion at the site of the injury. Except in instances of specific infections or trauma, which are largely preventable, good health may be directly ascribed to the maintenance of an erect position of the spine with all organ systems in equilibrium with it, and ill health may result from the alienation of organs or systems.

JOINT MEASUREMENTS

The Goniometer.—The goniometer is an instrument for measuring joint angles. This instrument consists of a half circle scale to which two long arms are attached by an axis pin to a level forming the diameter of the scale. Preferably a scale should be used which has two rows of figures from 0° to 180°, reading in opposite directions, so that in either direction a reading for motion is possible without changing the position of the instrument. The joint range is obtained by placing the protractor so that its axis pin is over the joint which is to be measured, with the upper arm of the instrument fixed parallel to the long axis of the segment above, and the lower arm of the protractor left free to move with the segment below the joint which is being measured.

A normal range of motion as established by the uninjured member should precede the measurement of the member in which there is restriction of movement. A reading is taken on the scale for the particular movement being measured, then recorded in degrees on the patient's record sheet. Motion is then made in the opposite direction and the reading is recorded again. The two readings constitute the normal range of motion; the number of degrees lacking in the same movement of the injured member constitutes the limitation of motion. The latter, or capacity range, should show a consecutive gain in amplitude consistent with treatment, the goal being the normal range as established by the normal member.

The patient's record sheet consists of a number of blank circle drawings or graphs on which the normal range is indicated in degrees, as well as the patient's capacity range and any subsequent gains in amplitude. The date of the first measurement may be placed on the record opposite the patient's capacity range for that time, and all later capacity ranges are likewise dated, thus providing an accurate record of the rate of progress by the patient.

Current Method of Joint Measurement.—At the present time, the usual method of measuring joint motion and restriction of movements is well illustrated by the following summary:

"Neutral position is that position of the joint from which measurements shall proceed. This may begin with readings on the scale indicated by 0°, 90°, 180°. Movements are measured either from 0° to 180° or 180° to 0°. Wherever the part stops in its course on the scale, the number opposite the part indicates the degree of motion. The number of degrees indicates the limitation of motion on the half circle scale and not the amount of motion. The zero end of the arc is toward the head and the median line of the body. As movement approaches the head, the angle of the joint becomes smaller, and the reading on the scale will be less. Motion away from the head will increase the angle, and the reading on the scale will go higher. The same is true when measuring toward and away from the body; the angle of motion will decrease as it approaches the median line and increases as it moves away from the median line. In rotation (including pronation and supination) the zero end is toward the median line of the body. Extension is toward 180°, whereas flexion is toward 0°, and the half circle arc is in the anteroposterior plane.

"Hyperextension is a movement toward the head and measurement will read from 180° to 0°. Adduction will read toward 0°, and abduction toward 180°. Internal rotation is toward 0°, and external rotation toward 180° on the anterior half circle in the transverse plane."[1]

Simplified Method of Joint Measurement.—It was found necessary to devise a more simplified method of measuring joint motion, one which would depict with a single reading the true amount of motion as obtained at that time. In the revised method of measuring joint motion, zero is established as that point in the scale at which there is the least amount of motion for the movement, and from which the particular movement shall proceed. The neutral point is that position in which the involved muscles are in equilibrium with their antagonists, and may be indicated in the scale as 0°, 90°, or 180°.

This system of measurement is in contradistinction to usual methods as depicted at the present time in literature, in which flexion is described as "that motion which approaches zero" and extension as "that motion which proceeds toward 360°."

[1] Krusen, Frank H., Physical Medicine, Philadelphia, W. B. Saunders Co., pp. 674, 1941.

In the current use of the goniometer, confusion may result when measuring extension of joints which pass the 180° point (hyperextension) and the reading has to be subtracted from 360°. In the simplified method of recording joint motion, this ambiguity is avoided and the full range of extension, as well as of any other motion, may be ascertained quickly and easily if the point at which the moving arm of the instrument stops indicates the exact amount of motion attained.

Examples of Joint Measurement Technique.—The following descriptions represent methods of measurements of the upper extremity; movements of the lower extremity are measured in a similar manner.

The accompanying graphs depict the recording of the joint measurement of both upper and lower extremities. (Figs. 1–6.)

Shoulder Joint Movements.—*Flexion.*—The goniometer is placed with the axis pin over the shoulder joint; the arm moves in the sagittal plane with the long axis of the humerus forward to a point above the head. The patient must be in either standing or sitting position for most shoulder joint movements; however, flexion may be taken in the supine position.

The movement of flexion proceeds from 0°, that position in which the arm is extended at the side. The normal range of the uninjured shoulder joint is first ascertained and recorded on a blank half circle record sheet as shown in the graphs. Then the injured member is likewise measured and recorded, the movement proceeding from 0°, moving forward and upward as far as it is able toward 180°, which is that position of the arm held straight above the head.

Extension.—This movement is performed in the same position and in the same plane as flexion, 0° being the point from which the movement is to begin; however, the arm is carried backward to its full capacity range. The movement is toward a theoretical 180° point backward and above the head. The normal and capacity ranges for both members are recorded and dated on the patient's graph.

Abduction.—Abduction is performed in a similar manner except that the arm is carried from the 0° position sideward in a frontal (coronal) plane. As it is anatomically possible to obtain only 90° abduction at the shoulder, movement above this and toward the 180° point above the head would include elevation also. The normal range for abduction-elevation in the frontal plane is 180°.

Adduction.—Adduction proceeds in the frontal plane from 0°, a position in which the arm is held sideward and extended high above the head in complete abduction-elevation. The arm moves sideward and downward toward the 180° point which is complete adduction of the arm at the side of the body. The technician is rarely required to measure this movement.

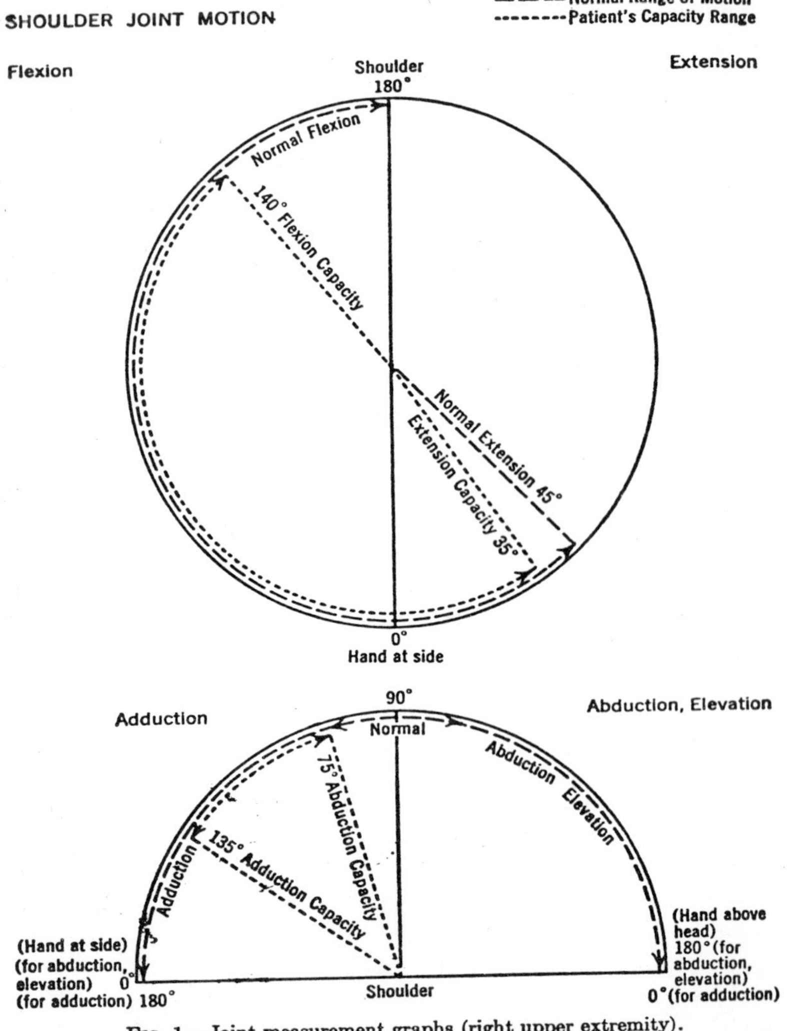

FIG. 1.—Joint measurement graphs (right upper extremity).

Elbow Joint Movements.—*Flexion.*—The goniometer is placed over the ulnar-humeral joint with the axis pin fixed over the joint, the stationary arm is parallel with the humerus, and the moving arm follows the midline of the forearm in flexion. The protractor may be placed either laterally or medially over the elbow joint, the forearm proceeding from the 0° position, which is that of complete extension of the elbow, and moving toward the shoulder to as full a range of flexion as is possible for the patient. One hundred and eighty degrees is that point toward which the arm moves.

Extension.—Restriction in extension is measured in the same fashion as flexion, except that the movement begins with a fully flexed position and proceeds toward the 180° position of complete

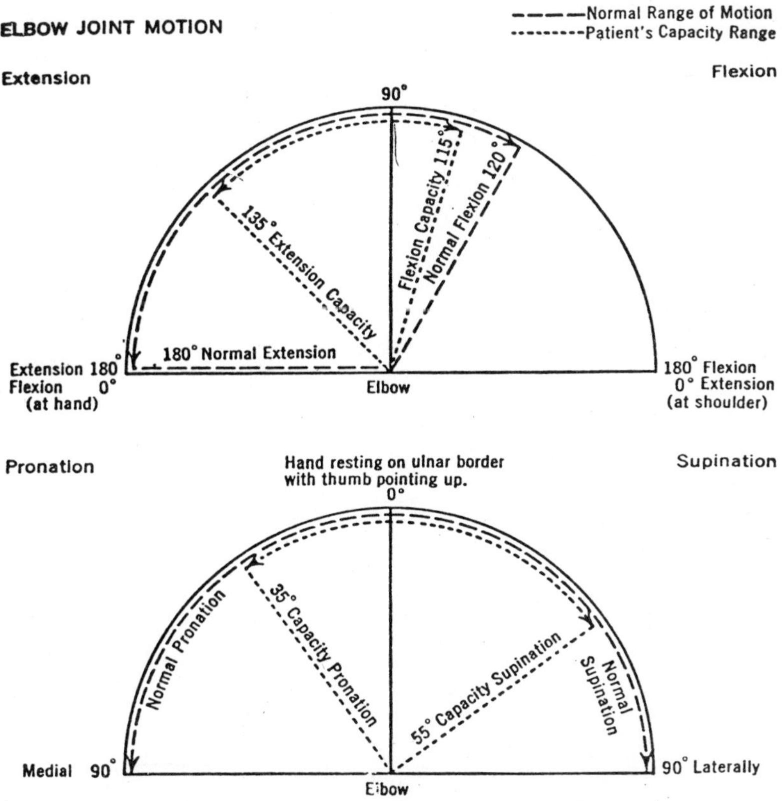

FIG. 2.—Joint measurement graphs (right upper extremity).

extension, which is the ordinary range for extension. Both movements may be made in sitting, standing, or recumbent position.

Supination and Pronation.—Both the movements are made with the elbow flexed, thumb pointing upward and proceeding from a 0° position, a neutral point in which supinators and pronators are in equilibrium. From this position of the forearm the movable arm of the protractor follows the hand as the forearm is turned lateralward in supination, or medialward in pronation. The point at which the movement of the arm stops will indicate in degrees the range of motion. Both normal and capacity ranges must be recorded for all movements.

Wrist Joint Movements.—Wrist motion is best performed with the patient seated, arm pronated and resting on a table while the hand is straight with the wrist extended over the opposite edge of the

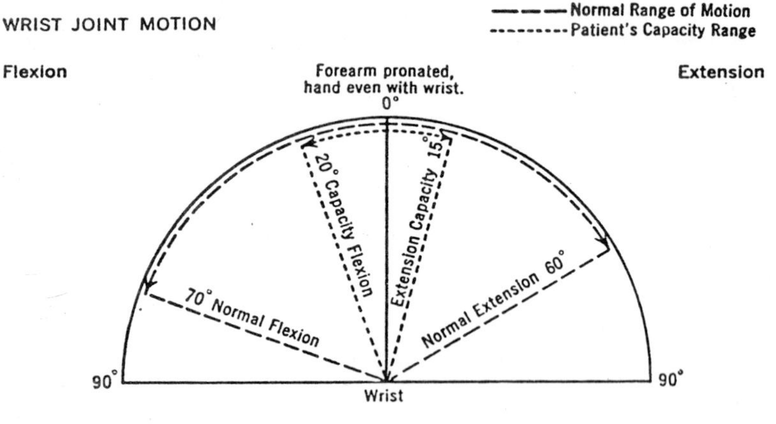

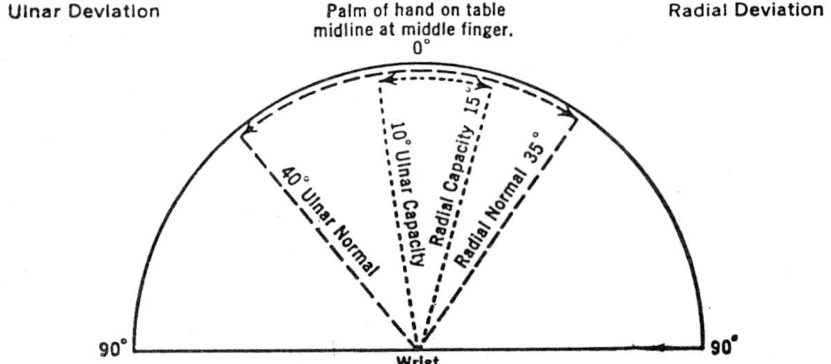

FIG. 3.—Joint measurement graphs (right upper extremity).

table and supported by the operator. This is a neutral position and may be designated as 0° for movements both of flexion and extension. The axis pin is placed over the styloid process of the ulna.

Flexion.—Flexion is ascertained by permitting the patient's hand to lower from the table edge as far as possible, the moving arm of the protractor following the ulna border of the hand to the capacity range, and a reading is taken.

Extension.—Extension is measured in the same manner except that the movement is upward to the full capacity range for extension. The complete capacity range for flexion-extension is the sum of the two ranges of motion.

Radial and Ulnar Deviations.—The elbow is flexed and the forearm is placed with the palm of the hand downward on a table for measurement of deviation at the wrist. The protractor is placed over the center of the wrist with the stationary arm fixed along the

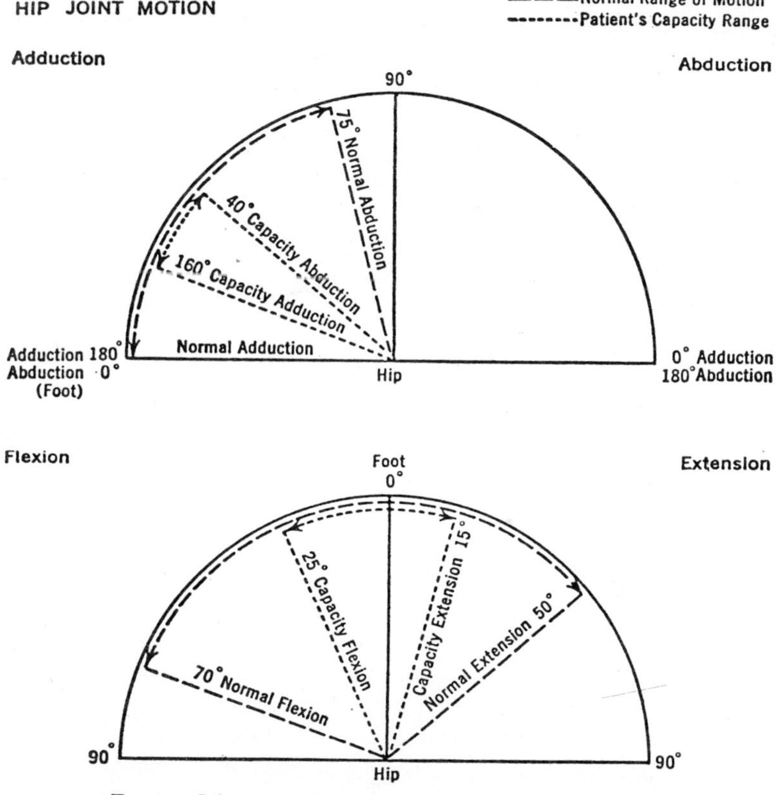

FIG. 4.—Joint measurement graphs (right lower extremity).

midline of the posterior forearm and the moving arm following medial (radial) and lateral (ulnar) movements as directed by the middle finger of the hand. The 0° position from which either movement proceeds is that point at the end of the middle finger when the hand is extended even with the wrist and pronated.

Indications for the Employment of the Goniometer.—There should be introduced some routine method of joint measurement in every physical medicine department for such cases as fractures, dislocations, sprains, arthritis or for any disability in which there are restrictions of movement. The joints should be measured regularly for determination of rates of progress and for permanent records[1] in litigation. In these cases measurements should be taken at the time of the first visit and at regular intervals thereafter, the normal range and all capacity ranges recorded and dated. Only in this manner is it possible for the physician following the case to obtain accurate estimation of the rate of progress of his patient.

Other Methods of Measuring Deficiencies of Joint Motion.—In case of ambiguity in attempting to evaluate disabilities by using

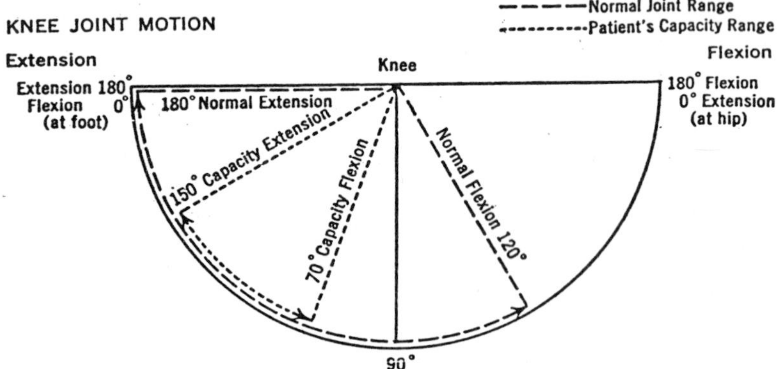

Fig. 5.—Joint measurement graphs (right lower extremity).

"degrees of motion" or "number of degrees" of limitation, other methods of describing the limitation of motion range may be substituted; for example, the attempt to evaluate restriction of "internal rotation" of the arm at the shoulder. It is very difficult to arrive at a definite measurement of limitation by goniometer reading as abduction, shoulder retraction, and pronation of the forearm complicate that of internal rotation. A restriction in internal rotation, however, may best be evaluated by a graphic description of just what movement the patient is able to perform, as his ability to place his thumb in his hip pocket, to place his hand at midline of his back at the level of his belt, or to raise his hand so that his thumb rests at the intra-scapular region. The same method may be used to describe the range of motion of other movements of the body and depict more clearly the situation.

[1] In all cases of disability in which there is litigation, it is important to have an accurate file of the joint measurements as obtained throughout the course of treatments so that a final degree of disability may be had before an adjustment is made if the part cannot be restored to normal function.

In the absence of a goniometer another method of measuring disability of a part is accomplished by using a piece of paper and placing the hand, arm or part to be measured upon the paper, then

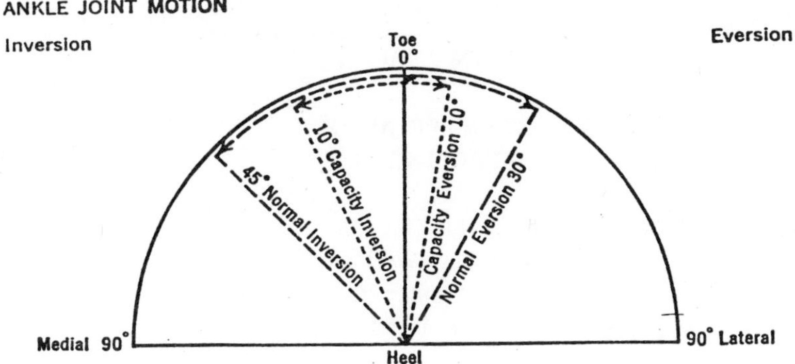

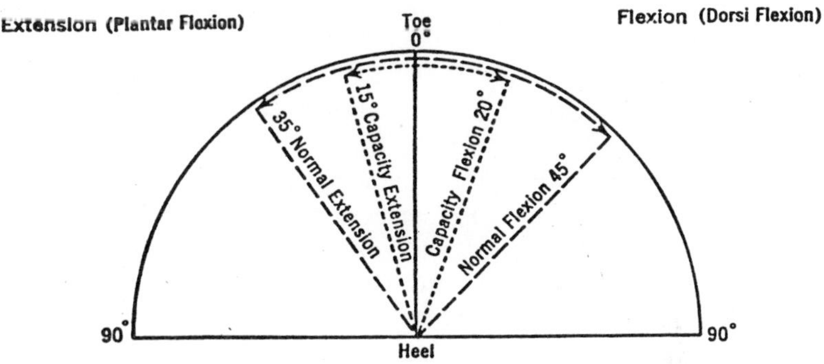

FIG. 6.—Joint measurement graphs (right lower extremity).

moving the segment to its capacity range and drawing an outline of the movement. In the same half-circle scale, draw in the line for the normal range for the individual as established by the uninjured member. Later drawings may be added as the patient gains in amplitude of capacity ranges, the newer ranges as well as all other ranges are dated to give a complete record of progress made as the injured member approaches the normal range, the dates implying the rate of progress.

CHAPTER III

BRIEF REVIEW OF MUSCLES PARTICIPATING IN JOINT MOVEMENTS

SKELETAL MUSCLES AS ORGANS OF THE MUSCULAR SYSTEM

Description of Muscles as Organs.—Skeletal muscles are not functionally separate and unrelated parts, but are grouped into a system which effects correlation and coöperation. Muscles never act singly (except when stimulated to perform isolated action by means of an electric current), but perform coöperatively to carry out a given act. We seldom contract a single muscle, but execute a movement in the performance of which several groups of muscles are involved.

By virtue of the activity of the voluntary muscles it is possible to maintain the posture characteristic of the species against the force of gravity. The manner in which the muscles are attached to the bony framework enables man to maintain erect posture, to hold his head erect; and muscular action results in movement and locomotion. Observation of everyday activity shows that there may be wide variations in extent of muscular movement. The skeletal muscles are adapted to carry out tasks of the utmost refinement, or are capable of performing tasks requiring large expenditure of energy.

Manner of Attachment of Muscles.—Each striated muscle consists of a body and two attachments. The body contains the muscular tissue; the attachments are composed of white fibrous tissue called tendons. The attachments of muscle to bone may be one of three types: direct to the periosteum, by means of an aponeurosis, or by means of a tendon. In the first, the connective framework of a muscle fuses with the fibrous layers of the periosteum of the bone; in the second, the aponeurosis is a flat heavy sheet of white fibrous tissue and connects muscle to bone or muscle to muscle; in the third, the connective tissue surrounding a muscle forming a band or cord extends to both ends of the muscle to attach it to the bones. The more fixed attachment of a muscle serves as the origin of action, the more movable attachment, where the effect of the motion is produced, is the insertion of the muscle.

If the attachments are known, its action may be determined by recalling that its insertion moves toward the origin when the muscle contracts in movement. Generally the origin is near the spinal axis of the body while the insertion is peripheral.

Arrangement of Muscles to Produce Motion.—Muscles are arranged in opposing or antagonistic groups. When muscles flexing a part are contracted, those opposing the action, the extensors, are in a state of physiological relaxation, in which they give way to the movement. Muscles which take the principal part in a specific joint movement are designated as prime movers, those aiding or controlling the specific movement are called synergists, and those which tend to oppose the specific movement are termed antagonists. Fixers are synergists which collaborate with the prime movers.

MUSCLES CONTROLLING THE PRINCIPAL JOINT MOVEMENTS IN THE UPPER EXTREMITY

Mechanism of the Shoulder Joint.—For a complete understanding of the kinesiology of the upper extremity it seems advisable to examine the mechanics of the joint.

A review of the movements of this, the most movable of all the joints in the body, shows a wide variety of movements which make possible the intricate and versatile mechanics displayed by man in his manual dexterity.

The joint is diarthrodial, lined by a synovial membrane, and contains synovial fluid. The synovial cavity almost always directly communicates with the bursa beneath the subscapularis muscle and sometimes with the one under the infraspinatus muscle. The articular capsule is a loose sac insufficient in itself to maintain the bones in contact; likewise, the ligaments are relatively weak.

The large spherical head of the humerus playing upon the shallow concave glenoid cavity of the scapula is retained in position much less by ligaments than by the muscles passing over the joint, and owing to the looseness of its capsule as well as to all the other conditions of its construction and position, it is exceedingly liable to be displaced. On the other hand, it is sheltered from violence by the projection of the acromion and the coracoid processes extending over it.

The scapula has no articulation with the axial skeleton but is joined with it indirectly through muscular attachments and through the clavicle.

The strength of the shoulder joint therefore lies in the powerful muscles passing over it, rather than in the ligaments holding the joint together. The synovial membrane sends a long tubular sheath to blend with the long head of the biceps muscle superiorly, and the articular capsule blends inferiorly with the origin of the triceps muscle.

Factors adding to the strength of the joint may be summed up as follows:

1. Tendons of muscles blending with the joint form part of the joint itself.
2. The muscles passing over the joint steadies the head of the humerus in its various movements.
3. These muscles help keep the head of the humerus against the glenoid cavity.
4. They also help by preventing the head of the humerus from gliding superiorly or inferiorly over the margin of the shallow glenoid cavity.
5. A shelf or vault is formed superiorly by the coraco-acrominal projections.
6. The mobility of the scapula is a factor in strengthening the shoulder joint, also the elasticity of the clavicle.
7. Atmospheric pressure aids the strength of the joint.
8. The strength of muscles passing over the joint offers a powerful restraining factor to the joint.

The weakness of the shoulder joint is readily explained by its free mobility, its exposure to injury, and the length of the humeral lever.

While dislocations are usually primarily subglenoid, owing to the lower part of the capsule being the thinner and less projected, they take usually a secondarily forward direction, as the triceps prevents the head passing backward. In addition, laxity of the lower part of the capsule is also a marked feature, allowing free abduction and elevation. These movements will be accordingly much checked by an inflammatory matting of this part of the capsule. Although the subdeltoid bursa does not communicate with the shoulder joint, it frequently becomes inflamed and may seriously interfere with movement of the shoulder joint. It may even become calcified. Rupture, partial or complete, of the tendon of the supraspinatus is of frequent occurrence, may involve the joint, and must be differentiated from subdeltoid or subacromial bursitis.

We feel that the space devoted to the description of the shoulder joint is justified here because of the relatively high incidence of injuries sustained by this joint, and because of the indication for physical medicine in many of these cases.

Review of Muscles Producing Motion of the Upper Extremity.— In a review of the muscles which take part in joint movement, it is unnecessary to state the origins and insertions, as the subject is primarily muscle action. However, students are required to locate the specific muscles on a skeleton in order to help visualize the movement which of necessity takes place from the location of the muscle. The muscles studied are organized into two groups:

1. Muscles arising chiefly from the scapula to move the humerus.
2. Muscles inserted into the scapula to produce the movements peculiar to that bone.

The following movements are given with the addition of the muscles participating in the movement and classified as to prime movers and synergists which aid in the movement:

Movements of the Scapula

Retraction

Prime Movers. Rhomboid Major
Rhomboid Minor
Trapezius

Synergists. Latissimus Dorsi

Protraction

Prime Movers. Serratus Anterior
Pectoralis Minor

Synergists. Upper portion of Pectoralis Major

Movements of the Humerus

Abduction

Prime Movers. Deltoid
Supraspinatus

When the arm is at the side the anterior and posterior fibers at the deltoid become adductors, but are abductors when the arm is being raised. The supraspinatus initiates the movement.

Synergists. Biceps (long head)
Infraspinatus

Adduction

Prime Movers. Pectoralis Major (lower part)
Latissimus Dorsi
Teres Major

Synergists. Triceps (long head)
Coracobrachialis
Biceps (short head)
Teres Minor

Extension

Prime Movers.	Latissimus Dorsi Deltoid (spinal portion)
Synergists.	Teres Major Subscapularis (when arm is at the side)

Flexion

Prime Movers.	Coracobrachialis (chief flexor)
Synergists.	Biceps (short head) Subscapularis (when arm is abducted)

Lateral Rotation

Prime Movers.	Infraspinatus (chief) Teres Minor
Synergists.	Posterior fibers of the deltoid

Medial Rotation

Prime Movers.	Subscapularis (chiefly) Latissimus Dorsi
Synergists.	All the adductors Anterior portion of deltoid (when arm is abducted) Biceps (long head)

The coracobrachialis, the scapular attachments of the triceps, and the biceps hold the humerus in the glenoid cavity.

Movements of the Forearm at the Elbow Joint.—Whereas the strength of the shoulder joint is maintained chiefly by tendons of muscles, the strength of the elbow joint is maintained chiefly by the bony structure of the elbow and the manner in which the humerus, radius and ulna articulate. The ligaments of the elbow joint, moreover, aid in its strength. The depth of the semilunar cavity and the perfect articulation of the olecranon process in the olecranon fossa posteriorly make it a strong bony union.

Movements of the Elbow.—Muscles acting on the forearm at the elbow.

Extension

Prime Movers.	Triceps Anconeus

Flexion

Prime Movers.	Brachialis Brachioradialis (supinator longus) Biceps (powerful when the arm is supinated)
Synergists.	Pronator Teres and Extensor Carpi Radialis Longus (strong) Flexor Carpi Radialis, Extensor Carpi Radialis Brevis, and Palmaris Longus (weak)

Supination

Prime Movers. Biceps
Supinator
Brachioradialis (only when the arm is extended and pronated)

Note: The brachioradialis and extensor carpi radialis longus bring the arm to an intermediate position. When the arm is extended, they supinate, but when the arm is flexed they become more and more pronators.

Pronation

Prime Movers. Pronator Teres
Pronator Quadratus

Synergists. Flexor Carpi Radialis

Movements of the Wrist.—The forms of the articular surfaces of the radiocarpal joint are those of an ellipsoidal diarthrosis; those of the intercarpal articulation are such as to permit modified hinge movement. The movements of these two anatomically separate articulations are combined in giving the hand its free motion at the wrist. The movements of the carpal articulation between bones of the same row are very limited and consist only of slight gliding upon one another; but slight as they are, they give elasticity to the carpus and break the jars and shocks which result from blows on the hand. All angular movements, including circumduction, are permitted in this combination of joints. The absence of rotation is compensated for by the movements of pronation and supination of the forearm. Flexion and extension occur around two axes, one for the radiocarpal, the other for the intercarpal, which pass obliquely from side to side through the capitate, close together. Abduction and adduction, or radial and ulnar flexion, as these movements are often named, take place about an antero-posterior axis through the capitate, and are contributed to by both the radiocarpal and the intercarpal articulations. Abduction is more limited than adduction and is checked by the ulnar collateral ligament and by contact of the styloid process of the radius with the greater multangular; adduction is checked by the radial collateral ligament alone.

Muscles acting on the wrist joint.

Extension

Prime Movers. Extensor Carpi Radialis Brevis
Extensor Carpi Radialis Longus
Extensor Carpi Ulnaris

Flexion

Prime Movers. Flexor Carpi Ulnaris
Flexor Carpi Radialis
Palmaris Longus

Note: The long flexor and extensors of the thumb and fingers are accessory flexors and extensors of the wrist. The long abductor of the thumb is also an accessory flexor of the wrist.

Radial Abduction

Prime Movers.	Extensor Carpi Radialis Longus Extensor Carpi Radialis Brevis
Synergists.	Abductor Pollicis Longus Extensor Pollicis Longus

Ulnar Abduction

Prime Movers.	Flexor Carpi Ulnaris Extensor Carpi Ulnaris

MOVEMENTS OF THE LOWER EXTREMITY AND MUSCLES PRODUCING ACTIONS

Movements of the Hip Joint—Its Clinical Weakness.—The hip joint, like the shoulder, is a ball and socket joint, but with much more complete socket and a corresponding limitation of movement. Each variety of movement is permitted—flexion, extension, abduction, adduction, circumduction, and rotation; any two or more of these movements not being antagonistic can be combined. Abduction and lateral rotation can be performed freely in every position of flexion and extension, abduction being limited by the pubocapsular ligament; lateral rotation by the iliofemoral ligament, especially its medial portion, during extension; but by the lateral portion, as well as by the ligamentum teres, during flexion. Adduction is very limited in the extended thigh on account of the contact with the opposite limb. In the slightly flexed position adduction is more free than in extension, and is then limited by the lateral fibers of the iliofemoral band and the superior portion of the capsule. In flexion the range is still greater and limited by the ischiocapsular ligament, the ligamentum teres being also rendered nearly tight. Medial rotation in the extended position is limited by the lower fibers of the iliofemoral ligaments and in flexion by the ischiocapsular ligament and the portion of the capsule between it and the iliofemoral band.

The articular cartilage (capsule) is one of the strongest ligaments in the whole body, but it is large and somewhat loose so that in every position of the body some portion of it is relaxed. Its thickness and strength vary greatly.

In the mid part and in the front of the capsule the iliopsoas bursa may communicate with the joint. This fact must be remembered in tuberculous disease of the psoas; the presence of this bursa explains certain deep-seated swellings in the front of the joint in adults, accompanied by a flexion contracture at the hip joint.

Dislocation usually occurs at the posterior, lower and medial part of the joint, as the circular and weaker part of the capsule is here. It should be noted that in full extension and flexion the head of the femur is in contact with the weakest spot in the capsule, in front and behind, respectively.

The following outlines the muscles which produce movement of the joint:

Extension

Prime Movers.	Gluteus Maximus
Synergists.	Adductor Magnus, and the Hamstrings (strong) Gluteus Medius, Piriformis, Obturator Internus (weak)

Flexion

Prime Movers.	Iliopsoas (chiefly) Pectineus
Synergists.	Rectus Femoris Adductor Longus and Brevis Obturator Externus Tensor Fasciæ Latæ Sartorius

Abduction

Prime Movers.	Tensor Fasciæ Latæ Gluteus Medius Gluteus Minimus
Synergists. (when joint is flexed)	Piriformis Obturator Internus Gemelli Sartorius

Adductors

Prime Movers.	Adductors Longus, Brevis, Magnus and Minimus Pectineus Obturator Externus
Synergists.	Gluteus Maximus and Quadratus Femoris (powerful in the standing position) Gracilis Obturator Internus

Note: With the thigh flexed at 90° angle:

Adduction—Iliopsoas
Abduction—Gluteus Maximus

Lateral Rotation

Prime Movers.	Quadratus Femoris Obturator Internus plus the Gemelli Obturator Externus Piriformis
Synergists.	Gluteus Maximus

Medial Rotation

Prime Movers.	Gluteus Medius Gluteus Minimus Tensor Fasciæ Latæ
Synergists.	Iliopsoas The adductors (except magnus)

Movements of the Knee Joint—Its Clinical Weakness.—The knee joint is the largest joint in the body. It is rightly described as a ginglymoid joint; but there are also other elements, for flexion and extension are modified by the spiral contour of the femoral condyles; in addition there is a sliding backward and forward of the tibia upon the femoral condyles, as well as slight rotation.

The knee is one of the most superficial and, because of the incongruity of the bony surfaces, one of the weakest joints; in no position are the bones in more than partial contact.

The strength of the knee lies in the number, size, and arrangement of the ligaments, and the powerful muscles and fascial expansions which pass over the articulation and enable it to withstand the leverage of the two longest bones in the body.

One of the most frequent traumas to the knee joint is that of lateral displacement. This is accounted for by the fact that the medial edge of the patella is more prominent, and thus more exposed to injury; it is also well supported, as is seen when the parts being relaxed, the fingers may be insinuated beneath each border. Also the pull of the quadriceps upon the patella, the ligamentum patellæ and the tibia is somewhat lateral. Movements of the knee joint are effected by these muscles acting to perform motions of the joint:

Extension

Prime Movers.	Quadriceps femoris	Rectus femoris Vastus externus, internus and intermedius
Synergists.	The tensor fasciæ latæ and the gluteus maximus acting through the ilio-tibial band help hold extended knee firm	

Flexion

Prime Movers.	The hamstring group Gracilis Sartorius Popliteus
Synergists.	Gastrocnemius

Movements of the Ankle Joint.—The ankle joint is a perfect ginglymus or hinge joint. The articulating bones are united by an articular capsule inclosing the joint cavity which is very extensive. Besides following the space inclosed within the articular capsule of the ankle, it extends upward between the tibia and fibula, forming a short cul-de-sac as far as the interosseus ligament. It is large in the anterior and posterior parts of the joint, and extends beyond the limits of the articulation, and is said to contain more synovial fluid than any other joint. Posteriorly the capsule is a very thin and disconnected membranous structure. However, the passage of the flexor hallucis tendon at the back materially strengthens the posterior part of the capsule. The main strength of the joint rests with the ligaments which pass over.

This being a true hinge joint, movements on one axis are the only ones permitted, there being no side-to-side motion, except in extreme extension. Flexion is limited by ligaments and the neck of the talus jutting over the edge of the tibia. Flexion and extension take place around a transverse axis drawn through the body of the talus.

Extension—Plantar flexion

Prime Movers.	Gastrocnemius and Soleus (triceps suræ) chiefly Peroneus Longus Tibialis Posterior Peroneus Brevis Flexor Digitorum Longus Flexor Hallucis Longus

Flexion

Prime Movers.	Tibialis Anterior Peroneus Tertius Extensor Hallucis Longus Extensor Digitorum Longus

Inversion—Supination

Prime Movers.	Tibialis Anterior
Synergists.	Tibialis Posterior Flexor Hallucis Longus

Eversion

Prime Movers.	Peroneus Longus Peroneus Brevis

Synergists. Peroneus Tertius
Extensor Hallucis Longus
Extensor Digitorum Longus

KINESIOLOGY OF THE SHOULDER GIRDLE AND ARM

Muscles of the Shoulder Girdle.—The following six muscles connect the shoulder girdle (clavicle and scapula) with the main skeleton, hold it in position, and give rise to movements involving the arm.

1. The trapezius muscle embraces four movements: lowers the back of the skull and turns it to one side, tending to lift the clavicle and scapula; tilts the acromion on the sternal end of the clavicle; pulls upon the spine of the scapula toward the spinal column; draws the vertrebral border of the scapula down and inward, toward the spine. All parts come into action at the same time in raising the arms sideward and especially in raising them above the shoulder level.
2. The levator scapulæ draws the scapula upward and inward as a whole rather than to rotate it.
3. The rhomboids adduct the lower angle of the scapula without the upper angle being adducted; they pull the scapula downward.
4. The serratus magnus draws the scapula forward as a whole without rotation. The lower part of the muscle is in a position to produce vigorous rotation upward by drawing the inferior angle of the scapula forward. It is to be noted how well these lower fibers are placed to associate with the trapezius in turning the glenoid fossa upward.
5. The pectoralis minor is the antagonist of the rhomboids It draws the scapula forward and somewhat downward.
6. The subclavius depresses the clavicle and draws it inward. It strengthens its joint with the sternum.

ELEVATION OF THE ARM

It is noticed that certain movements of the arm involve not only motion of the shoulder joint, but also motion in the shoulder girdle; therefore, it is necessary to study carefully the action of the six muscles which perform movements of the shoulder girdle.

It is found that when the arm is moved in any of its four cardinal directions, the shoulder joint itself is moved in a position most favorable for the movement; also, the glenoid fossa, by the gliding of the scapula over the surface of the chest or a rotation upward or downward, is brought into position so as to face in either upward or downward direction. Then the scapula is firmly anchored to the trunk so as to make the glenoid fossa a solid fulcrum from which the arm may swing as a lever.

Normal elevation of the arm is a movement from rest at the patient's side through 180° and its return to rest in a vertical position. To raise the arm to a vertical position requires movement in the shoulder joint and upward rotation of the scapula. The mechanics of this movement follow: In abduction elevation the humerus is first moved in the shoulder joint without any considerable movement of the scapula through from 10° to 45° by the action of the middle deltoid and the supraspinatus, while the entire trapezius, excepting the clavicular fibers, contracts to prevent the scapula from being rotated downward by the weight of the arm. During the next 90° of elevation both the scapula and the humerus are moving, the lower serratus acting to swing the lower angle of the scapula forward. In completion of the movement, the upper 45° of elevation takes place in the shoulder joint only. At about the time the arm passes the horizontal, the anterior fibers of the deltoid begin to act to aid the middle part, and the upper trapezius also contracts. When elevation is sideward, the arm must be rotated outward, preferably when near the shoulder level, to prevent the locking of the joint by contact of the bones at the top of the vault.

One theory contends that when the arm has reached the 90° angle, the humerus meets the bony block of the coraco-acromial vault, and that for the arm to be brought overhead in a vertical position, the scapula must be tilted upward so that the humerus may then swing upward without interference of the bony projection over it.

RE-EDUCATION OF THE UPPER EXTREMITY

(*A*) ELEVATORS OF THE SHOULDER GIRDLE

Trapezius (upper part), and levator anguli scapulæ

Position 1

The patient sits erect with the arm hanging at the side, and raises the shoulder as high as possible.

(*a*) With the resistance of gravity alone.

(*b*) With the added resistance of the physician's hand pressing down on the point of the shoulder.

(*B*) ABDUCTORS OF THE UPPER ARM

Deltoid, supraspinatus and biceps
plus
The muscles which turn the scapula so that the glenoid fossa points upward (trapezius and serratus magnus)

Position 1

The patient lies on his back with the arm at the side and moves it sideways upward along the table until it is stretched above his head.

(*a*) With assistance under the elbow.
(*b*) Without outside help.
(*c*) With resistance above the elbow.

Position 2

The patient sits erect with the arm at the side and raises it straight sideward until it is stretched vertically above his head.

(*a*) With the resistance of the weight of the arm.
(*b*) With the added resistance of the physician's hand pushing down just above the elbow.

If it is desired to exclude movement of the scapula in the preceding exercises, the physician must hold the shoulder girdle down firmly with one hand, in which case the arm will be raised only to shoulder height.

Any loss of power in the deltoid is apt to be more permanent than loss of power in other muscles, so that its training is often very discouraging.

(*C*) ADDUCTORS OF THE UPPER ARM

Pectoralis major, latissimus dorsi and teres major
plus
The muscles which turn the scapula so that the glenoid fossa points downward (rhomboideus major and minor, and pectoralis minor)

Position 1

The patient lies on his back with the arm stretched above his head, and moves it sideways downward along the table until it touches the side.

(*a*) With the assistance above the elbow.
(*b*) With the resistance of the friction of the table.
(*c*) With the resistance of the physician's hand below the elbow.

Position 2

The patient sits with the arm stretched vertically above the head and brings the arm sidewise downward to the body, while the physician gives resistance on the under side of the arm just above the elbow.

This exercise may be used for either very weak or very strong adductors, according to the amount of resistance given.

To exclude movement of the scapula in the preceding exercises the physician must hold the shoulder girdle down firmly, in which case the starting position will be with the arm at shoulder height.

(*D*) THE MUSCLES WHICH MOVE THE UPPER ARM FORWARD

Pectoralis major (upper part), deltoid (anterior part), coracobrachialis and biceps

plus

The muscles which turn the scapula so that the glenoid fossa points upward (trapezius and serratus magnus)

Position 1

The patient lies on one side with the opposite arm straight and lying against the side and raises this arm straight upwards until it is stretched above his head.

(*a*) With assistance on the back of the elbow.
(*b*) Without outside help.
(*c*) With resistance on the front of the elbow.

Care must be taken that the patient does not roll and fling the arm.

Position 2

The patient sits erect with the arm at the side and raises it straight forward upwards until it is stretched vertically above his head.

(*a*) With the resistance of the weight of the arm.
(*b*) With the added resistance of the physician's hand pushing on the front of the elbow.

To exclude movement of the scapula, the physician must hold the shoulder girdle down firmly and allow the arm to be raised to shoulder height only.

(*E*) FLEXORS OF THE FOREARM ON THE UPPER ARM

Biceps, brachialis anticus, supinator longus or brachioradialis, pronator radii teres, flexor carpi radialis, flexor carpi ulnaris, palmaris longus and flexor sublimis digitorum

Position 1

The patient sits with the under side of the whole arm resting on a table and bends the elbow by sliding the forearm along the surface of the table.

(*a*) With assistance on the back of the wrist.
(*b*) With resistance on the front of the wrist.
(*c*) By unaided contraction of the muscles.

Care must be taken that the patient does not perform the movement by creeping with the fingers on the table.

Position 2

The patient sits with the elbow resting on a cushion and raises the forearm until the hand touches the shoulder.

(*a*) With the resistance of gravity alone.
(*b*) With added resistance on the front of the wrist.

(*F*) EXTENSORS OF THE FOREARM ON THE UPPER ARM

Triceps, anconeus, extensor carpi ulnaris, and extensor communis digitorum

The positions for the exercises are the same as for the flexors of the forearm, but the exercises themselves are exactly the reverse.

(*G*) OUTWARD ROTATORS OF THE FOREARM

Biceps, supinator longus (brachioradialis), and supinator brevis

Position 1

The patient sits with the arm supported on the table, elbow flexed and palm down, and turns the hand over until the palm is facing upwards. The brachioradialis with the arm extended, supinates the forearm.

Position 2

The physician grasps the patient's hand (as if to shake hands) and offers resistance as the patient turns the hand over.

(*H*) INWARD ROTATORS OF THE FOREARM

Pronator radii teres, pronator quadratus, supinator longus (brachioradialis), and flexor carpi radialis

The exercises are exactly the reverse of those for the outward rotators of the forearm.

RE-EDUCATION OF THE LOWER EXTREMITY

In the case of re-educating muscles of the lower extremity the use of the roller skate or a ball bearing device attached to a shoe reduces friction and has been found an advantage in facilitating early motion. This contrivance has been found very helpful in fractures of the lower extremity. With the ball bearing under the heel and the lift under the knee, regulated by the patient himself, the gentlest movements in flexion and extension can be executed, just as much assistance being given as the case may require without danger of injury if ordinary care is used. Resistance in the nature of push and pull by an attendant may be added. This arrangement provides for flexion and extension of both knee and hip as well as for abduction and adduction of the hip. Abduction and adduction are provided for by turning the wheels fixed at right angles to the shoe. This type of exercise will be found useful in practically all types of fracture of the lower extremity, including especially fracture of the patella and fracture of the neck of the femur where special care is indicated.

There is probably little doubt that some potentially good results after fracture of the neck of the femur are ruined by too early removal of apparatus in bed. The strain at the fracture site, from the constant tendency of the thigh and foot to rotate out, represents a force that probably results frequently in a gradual giving way of the soft callus with the result of a fibrous union. Instructions to the patient to move the leg in bed in the sense of abduction and adduction, or, worse still, to try to lift the heel from the bed with the knee extended, can be detrimental as these movements cause tremendous force to come into play, tending to angulate the neck of the femur into a position of coxa vara. In a leg slightly edematous still greater caution is indicated because of increased weight. Because of muscle pull this internal stress on the bone is very considerable as has been demonstrated. It is more than likely that attention to details of this character help to cut down the percentage of failure in fractures of the neck of the femur and to reduce the healing period in this as well as other fractures of the lower extremity.

Conditions in which sling suspension may be employed with benefit include spastic paralysis, especially of the lower extremities, and atrophic arthritis, as well as in cases of weakness and stiffness after fracture or injury. In spastic paralysis it has frequently been found of advantage to attach a heavy weight to the sling, transforming it essentially into a pendulum with heavy weight. The patient's arm or leg is placed in the sling and the pendulum is put into motion by the instructor, the patient being taught to continue the swinging with and without resistance. It is felt that a good start may be made in this manner in developing the sense of rhythm and in the teaching of gentle coördinate movement.

In arthritis, non-weight-bearing active motion within the pain-free range is without doubt a factor of considerable importance in the maintenance of normal physiologic joint activity. The alternate contraction and relaxation of muscle groups and their antagonists must be of help in improving the circulation. As the muscles contract, the lymph vessels and veins are compressed, the blood and lymph being hurried in the proximal direction. In this manner capillary stasis is overcome with definite acceleration of the blood stream resulting. All the tissues of the part, including those of the joint, are benefited by the improved circulation. Cell growth, repair, and defense, as well as elimination, are enhanced. It is felt that the use of the ball bearing apparatus in atrophic arthritis is of special value, since, with the apparatus in place, the patient can exercise frequently for brief periods, always in the pain-free range. Practically all the joints of the lower extremity and those of the upper extremity as well are brought into play, the latter through the rope and pulley hand control.

CHAPTER IV

PHYSIOLOGY OF SKELETAL MUSCLE

HISTOLOGICAL STRUCTURE OF MUSCLE FIBER

An understanding of the microscopic structure of skeletal muscle increases a comprehension of muscular performance and lays a good foundation for a more complete conception of, and skill in adminstering, therapeutic exercise. For this reason we will consider the striated or skeletal muscle only, as we are studying voluntary muscular action.

A muscle is an organ composed of many thousands of muscle fibers bound together by connective tissue and surrounded by a sheath of the same tissue.

Muscle tissue is composed of cells which are designated by various names; such as fibers, sarcomere, or sarcostyle. Each fiber, or unit of structure is a many nucleated minute, cylindrical or prismatic thread whose diameter varies perhaps between 0.1 and 0.01 millimeter and whose length depends on the size and shape of the muscle. These are the muscle cells bound together by connective tissue into larger masses forming the muscle. Each fiber is ensheathed by a delicate membrane called the sarcolemma; running through its entire length are a great number of fine parallel filaments, the myofibrils, which are embedded in the sarcoplasm within the fiber. The myofibrils consist of alternating dim and light disks or segments, which when falling together in the different fibrils give cross striations, characteristics of skeletal muscles. In each fiber these myofibrils are grouped together in bundles (sarcostyles) with scanty sarcoplasm between. The myofibrils are the contracting units of the fibers and therefore of the muscle, as the contractile power of a muscle depends upon the combined effect of the innumerable fibers of which it is composed. The sarcoplasm is the nutritive factor. The myofibrils contain the transverse bands which give the skeletal muscles their characteristic appearance or striated effect, because they exhibit dim and light bands (which are designated below by different letters). Occurring at regular intervals along the fibril and dividing it into a series of compartments or sarcomeres, are Krause's membranes. In each sarcomere are dark areas, the dim or Q bands, and on either side lighter areas, the light or J bands. All myofibrils are composed of similar sarcomeres, containing light and dim bands in the proportion of two J bands and one Q band.

HISTOLOGY OF MUSCULAR CONTRACTION

In contraction, the phenomenon takes place within the fibril, the sarcomere becoming shortened in the long diameter and thickened in cross diameter. The mechanism of the dim and light bands in a single sarcomere explains the visible alterations which also take place in thousands of other sarcomeres. It is thought that there is a splitting asunder of the two dim Q bands, the two halves moving away from each other and from the Q band center (M) as far as the limiting telophragma (Krause's membrane). This effect repeated in all fibrils causes a shortening of the muscle as a whole. The entire phenomenon, though not well understood, is explained on the hypothesis that the dim (Q) or anisotrophic bands consist of a doubly refractive substance, whereas the light bands (J) or isotrophic bands are singly refractive (like water or glass). Those doubly refractive bands have the power to split two ways, as their appearance by polarized light.

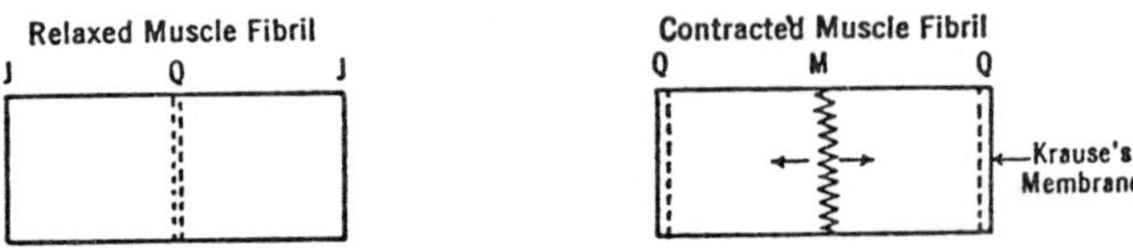

FIG. 7.—Graph depicting contractile phase of muscle fibril.

TYPES OF STRIATED MUSCLES AND METHODS OF ATTACHMENT

There are red and white muscles thought to be differentiated by rapidity of contraction. The white have more striations; the red are smaller, have more granules and slower contractions.

The fibers or muscle cells vary considerably in length and are arranged differently in the various muscles; *e. g.*, unipenniform, bipenniform, multipenniform, and fusiform. In general they are bound together in bundles by a fascia covering the entire muscle and often dividing the muscle into subdivisions. The elongation of the muscle covering extends to form the tendons of insertion and origin. This connective tissue covering, which is especially developed at the end of the fibers, serves to attach them either directly to the structure on which the muscle acts or to the skeletal framework of the muscle. In a few cases they may attach directly to the periosteum and very infrequently to an aponeurosis. Each fiber has its blood supply from a nearby capillary, there being a network of capillaries throughout the muscle.

PROPERTIES OF MUSCLE

To the fibril we owe all the properties of muscle, conductivity, elasticity, irritability, and contractility. Muscular tissue when acted upon by a weight extends quite readily, but on removal of the weight regains its original form by reason of its elasticity. In dead elastic bodies the strain is proportional to the stress, whereas in living tissue the strain and extension are not proportional to the weight used. A muscle is composed of viscous material and yields to the force acting upon it.

A muscle has the power of independent irritability, as shown by its reaction of contraction when artificial stimuli is applied directly to its tissue substance, even after its complete degeneration when the nerve has been cut. It is able to maintain or exert tension on its origin and insertion only because of its intact nerve supply This is called muscle tonus.

PHYSIOLOGY OF MUSCLE CONTRACTION

Effect of Artificial Stimuli.—Muscles may be made to contract by various agents; such as heat, mechanical factors, chemical factors, and electrical stimulation.

Not only is heat a possible cause of muscle contraction, but also it is an effect. Initial or anaerobic heat is that heat energy liberated during contraction. Aerobic or delayed heat is heat released during the period of recovery when oxygen is required. The caloric increase can be calculated as follows:

Weight of muscle	=	20 m.
Rise in temperature	=	.005 calories
Specific heat of muscle	=	.83
20 m. × .83 × .005	=	calories produced

The electrical stimulus is found to be very practical because it can be readily controlled as to intensity and affects all fibers simultaneously, giving coördinated contraction of all fiber bundles. The normal stimulus for muscle contraction in the body is found to be chemical in nature; and the effect of the nerve fiber upon muscle fiber is conveyed through a chemical transmitter by way of a myoneural junction.

Simple contraction of muscle resulting from one stimulus varies in reaction time; the same stimulus requires 0.1 second in the frog and 0.01 second in mammals.

Types of Contraction.—In an isotonic contraction there is a change in length, an actual contraction, and the load is equal to the capacity.

In an isometric contraction there is no change in length; the load is more than the capacity.

Factors Affecting Contraction.

(1) *Strength of Stimuli.*

(*a*) Minimal contraction: the stimulus is just enough to produce a visible contraction.

(*b*) Subminimal contraction: there is less stimulus than for minimal contraction.

(*c*) Maximum contraction: the stimulus increases until no further stretching is possible on additional stimuli.

(*d*) Sub-maximal contraction: contraction between (*a*) and (*c*).

(2) *Effects of Temperature.*

0° C — entire loss of irritability.

5° to 9° C — maximum irritability and greatest contracture.

15° to 18° C — gradual decrease of contracture.

26° to 30° C — second maximum, greater or less than first.

37° C — entire loss of irritability.

Contractures.—A prolonged condition of shortening from a single stimulus produces sometimes a state of contracture (a maintained state of retarded relaxation).

Rapidly repeated contractions produce the following effects:

(*a*) The first three or four introductory contractions decrease in extent.

(*b*) Treppe is an increase in contractions with constant stimuli.

(*c*) Fatigue appears after repeated "treppe" and the muscle fails to react to stimuli because of a loss of irritability resulting from repeated activity and a consequent accumulation in the tissue of fatigue products.

All or None Law.—When a muscle fiber contracts in response to nerve impulse, which stimulates sufficiently to produce action, it contracts to its fullest extent. This applies to the motor unit alone and not to the entire muscle. The number of units acting and the rhythm with which they act contribute to the variations in the strength of a contraction. If the motor units are acting synchronously, there is a better contraction than when they are responding asynchronously. The contraction wave starts at a point of stimulus and spreads over the fiber wi'' a definite velocity. As more fibers are involved, the muscle is tnen capable of a greater contraction.

Efficiency of Muscle as a Work Machine.—The amount of work is calculated directly by the amount of heat given off and indirectly by the amount of material consumed.

Q = total energy developed from material consumed
W = work done
E = efficiency

$$\frac{W}{Q} = E$$

Work is performed by the shortening of the muscle because of the utilization, in some way, of the original chemical energy potential developed which does not take the form of heat.

The Curve of Work and Absolute Power of a Muscle.—The absolute power of a muscle is reached with the maximum tension without any alteration of its natural length.

The curve of work is estimated:

1. No work is done if no weight is lifted.
2. The optimum load for each muscle is reached when the greatest unit of work is done.
3. If the load is enough to counteract the contraction, there is no work done.

Measurements show that the absolute power of frog muscle per sq. cm. cross area is 0.7 Kg. to 3 Kg.; that of human muscle per sq. cm. cross area is 6.24 Kg.

Work done for any muscle is increased by increasing the length of the fibers, by greater tension, or by increasing the load.

Compound or Tetanic Contractions.—There is a complete compound or tetanic contraction if there is a fusion of contractions resulting from separate stimuli or if the total shortening is greater than that caused by maximal contraction. There is incomplete compound or tetanic contraction if the rate is not rapid enough, as there is a relaxation after each stimulus; or it may be incomplete by numerous degrees, according to the rates of stimuli. A muscle in tetanus remains in contraction as long as stimuli are sent into it.

Summation occurs when the total shortening of the muscle in tetanus may be considerably greater than that caused by maximal simple contractions. Fusion of contractions is due to the accruing of separate stimuli.

There is a discontinuous character of tetanic contractions, though the contractions seem continuous. That each stimulus has its own effect can be shown, but the chemical changes underlying the phenomena are known to be of an uninterrupted character.

The number of stimuli necessary for complete tetanus varies with the kind of muscle and the rapidity of the process of relaxation shown by the muscle in simple contraction. Contracture tetanus may become complete on account of retarded relaxation because of maintained stimuli.

The Phenomenon of Muscle Tone.—On stimulation of a muscle directly or through its motor nerve, one may hear through the stethoscope a muscial note given off corresponding in pitch to the number of stimuli given.

Muscle Tonus and Postural Sense -All muscles with intact nerve supply in a conscious individual maintain a continuous state of slight contraction. This mild contraction, sustained because of the reflex stretching of the muscle owing to the pull between its attachments, is accounted for by the fact that only a few motor units are working and do so in continual rotation. Tonus is greatest in states of excitement and positions of readiness, lower in normal standing and sitting positions, and progressively less in relaxation, rest positions, and sleep.

Muscle tonus is a condition of tension or contraction independent of voluntary innervation. It is a reflex phenomenon due to a mild stretch of the muscle between its attachments and is neurogenic rather than myogenic; the initial cause lies in the nervous system and not in the muscle itself. There is a loss of tone if afferent nerves are cut in the posterior roots of the spinal cord.

Tonus is the result of a number of factors as enumerated below:

1. Tonus is the result of proprioceptor cells in tendons, muscles, and joints.
2. Tonus may occur as a result of stimulus by cold.
3. Tonus maintains posture of the head as a result of sensory apparatus of the bony labyrinth of the middle ear.

Tonus "neurogenis" is the normal tonus of the body muscles coming from the central nervous system and not from the muscle itself. It is a reflex phenomenon connected with the maintenance of posture. Tonus involved with involuntary control and arising in tendons, joints, or muscles (proprioceptor cells) causes tonic hardening of the muscles and fixation of joints necessary for the standing position. This reflex is developed by the stretch of the muscle tendon mechanically between its points of attachments.

Theories of Tonus and Contraction.—Botazzio[1] believed that ordinary contraction is mediated by the fibrils and that tonic contraction is a reaction in the sarcoplasm between the fibers.

Bolzer[1] believed that there are two kinds of fibrils in each fiber: the tetanus or twitch fibrils lying next to the sarcolemma, and the tonus fibrils (smaller and less easily stained) lying in the central portion of the fiber.

[1] Howell, William H.: Physiology for Medical Students and Physicians, 14th Ed., Philadelphia, W. B. Saunders Co., 1941.

The usual view is that both ordinary contraction and tonus are the same and are affected through the neuromuscular mechanism. In tonic contraction, fewer fibers and units are in action at any one time, frequency of stimulation is lower (5 to 7 per second) giving a feebler contraction.

Voluntary Contractions.—A voluntary contraction is a neuromuscular mechanism involving the *higher centers* and subject to the will. Most voluntary contractions are too long to be simple contractions. There is direct evidence obtained by experimentation which records the number of complete contractions which enter into the production of voluntary tetanus. There is indicated a slow rate of rhythm approximating a rate of twenty stimuli per second. Questions as to whether a simple as well as a compound contraction may be elicited voluntarily have been answered by direct investigation. It is shown that even the shortest possible voluntary contractions are brief tetani made up of a short, lasting series of contractions fused together. In all probability, therefore, the motor centers, whenever they are stimulated by a so-called act of the will, discharge rhythmically a series of nerve impulses.

One theory of the mechanism of muscular contraction is that a muscle is a chemo-dynamic engine in which chemical energy is converted to mechanical work without passing through the form of heat. However, there is no evidence to explain the act of shortening. This theory along with many others is no longer accepted. Now it is believed that the myofibril, composed mainly of myosin, is made up of chains of polypeptids with their long axis to the long axis of fibrils bound by linkages between terminal groups. These fibrils show configuration corresponding to dim and light bands, the first of which show double refraction and are parallel to the long axis; the latter are folded, are at an angle, and have weak double refraction. Contraction may be due to folding and to superfolding of the myosin molecular chain which is rapidly reversed at relaxation.

There is an instrument called the Ergograph which is used to record voluntary contractions. If rest and load are kept constant, the test shows the following results:

1. There is no fatigue if there is sufficient rest between contractions.
2. A long rest of at least two hours is needed for the second test after the muscle has been completely fatigued.
3. After complete fatigue, effort to further contract the muscle greatly prolongs the recovery period.
4. Local or general lack of nutrition affects and diminishes the power of the muscle.
5. Improved nutrition increases power to do work.

6. The total amount of work done is greater with small loads than with large loads.
7. Marked activity in one set of muscles diminishes power in other muscles.

Muscular Sensibility.—There is an abundance of afferent nerve supply to muscles. The motor fibers are mixtures of afferent and efferent fibers. Some of the afferent fibers which are connected with definite receptor organs within the muscle and the muscle spindles in this way initiate a reflex contraction within the muscle. The muscle spindles are the receptor organs in the muscle which regulate the reflex control of the limbs.

Muscle Sense.—Muscular contraction or muscular tension gives rise to consciousness of the state of contraction of the muscle or the degree of flexion or extension of the limb. Through this mechanism are regulated our voluntary movements.

Pressure Sense.—This phenomenon is present still after the cutaneous nerves in the skin have been severed and is aroused by a force acting downward through the skin.

The Relation of the Chemical Changes During Contraction to Fatigue.—Fatigue, a condition of loss of irritability and contractility, is brought about by functional activity. Experiments on frogs show that extracts from fatigued muscle of one, when injected into the circulation of a second, brought on fatigue in the latter's muscles. These substances were proved by Hanke[1] to be the known products of muscular metabolism. Violent exercise may cause an accumulation in the blood of lactic acid, showing that such a large increase indicates that the oxygen supply to the contracting muscle is inadequate. Therefore, muscles may acquire an accumulated oxygen debt owing to the ability of the muscle to give more or less anaerobic contractions. The resulting pile-up of lactic acid may enter the blood stream and diminish the amount of work that other unused muscles may do.

The phenomenon of Treepe[1] is explained thus as the increased irritability caused by the first effects of the fatigue substance; later effects of the substance diminish the irritability or suppress it altogether. Fatigue, therefore, is mainly caused by an accumulation of lactic acid and may develop while the muscle still contains energy-yielding material.

Fatigue Sense.—This mechanism serves as a check to prevent overstrain of muscles, and may pass into a state of pain. These pain-producing substances, possibly lactic acid, are bodies formed

Howell, William H.: Physiology for Medical Students and Physicians, 14th Ed., Philadelphia, W. B. Saunders Co., 1941.

in the chemical changes of contraction. In excessive muscular effort the chemical substances escape into the circulation and tend to lower the threshold of painful sensibility in other muscles including probably the heart.

The Effects of Exercise on Condition of Muscles.—Muscles will atrophy on disuse and failure of the nerve supply, as well as by means of any alteration in the normal metabolism. A good muscle, therefore, is a used muscle. The increase in size of muscles is due to an increase in volume and not to an increase in the number of fibers. Artificial stimulation by electricity causes better nutrition as the store of glycogen is markedly increased thereby. Factors due to exercise which influence the nutrition of a muscle are those which will tend to increase the circulatory supply. Tonus is necessary to normal nutrition of the muscle.

CHEMISTRY OF MUSCULAR CONTRACTION

The isolated muscle derives the energy for its contraction ultimately from the combustion of carbohydrate. Oxygen is consumed and carbon dioxide produced. The actual contraction of the muscle, however, is brought about by the explosive breakdown of a non-carbohydrate compound called phosphocreatine into creatine and phosphoric acid.

There are two phases concerned in the chemistry of muscular contraction, the non-oxidative or anaerobic phase in which no oxygen is needed, and the oxidative, recovery or aerobic phase. Following relaxation, one-fifth of the lactic acid produced during the contraction is oxidized; the energy derived from this reaction is utilized in the resynthesis of the remaining four-fifths of the lactic acid to glycogen. The intermediate step in the breakdown of glycogen to lactic acid is the formation of fructose diphosphate; that is, a sugar containing six carbon atoms combined with two molecules of phosphoric acid. The carbon dioxide is received by the blood stream and excreted by the lungs. The lactic acid, partly neutralized within the muscular tissue by buffer salts and partly changed back into glycogen for future use involving the production of heat, gives the characteristic feeling of warmth after activity.

As no carbon dioxide is formed when a stimulus reaches a muscle, and as the change responsible for the energy of shortening is not an oxidation because the carbon dioxide is produced after the contraction is over, the amount of carbon dioxide produced is *just* the index of the amount of carbohydrates or fat oxidized. The whole process is concerned with restoration of energy to the muscle and not an index of the energy used in the contraction itself.

CHAPTER V

PLEXUSES OF NERVES CONTROLLING THE UPPER AND LOWER EXTREMITIES

THE BRACHIAL PLEXUS OF THE UPPER EXTREMITY

Introduction: Schematic Drawing and Word Picture of the Formation of the Brachial Plexus.—*Stage 1:* Anterior primary divisions of the fifth, sixth, seventh, eighth cervical, and first thor-

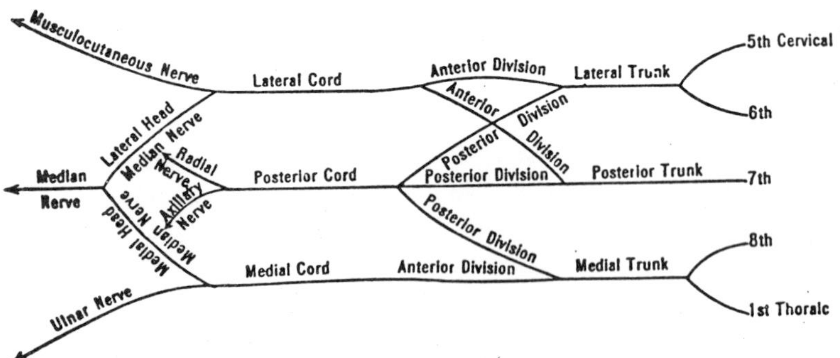

Fig. 8.—Word picture of the formation of the brachial plexus.

acic nerves, occasionally slips from the fourth cervical and second thoracic. The divisions unite to form the trunks of the brachial plexus.

Stage 2: The anterior primary divisions unite to form three trunks: the lateral trunk is formed from the fifth and sixth cervical; the middle trunk, from the seventh cervical nerve; the lower trunk, from the eighth cervical and the first thoracic.

Stage 3: Each trunk has anterior and posterior divisons which go to form the cords of the brachial plexus.

Stage 4: Anterior divisions from the lateral and middle trunk of the fifth, sixth, seventh cervical nerves unite to form the lateral cord. Posterior divisions from the three trunks of the fifth, sixth, seventh, eighth cervical and the first thoracic unite to form the posterior cord. Anterior division from the lower trunk of the eighth cervical and the first thoracic nerves forms the medial cord.

Stage 5: Terminal branches from the three cords give off branches which form the nerves of the arm, forearm, and hand. The lateral cord gives off the musculocutaneous nerve and the lateral component of the median nerve.[1] The posterior cord terminates in two branches, the radial nerve (musculospiral), and the axillary nerve (circumflex). The anterior cord gives off the ulnar nerve and the medial component of the median nerve. The lateral or outer head of the lateral cord and the medial or inner head of the medial cord unite to form the median nerve.

The picture presented above is merely to give the student in physical therapy a diagrammatic outline of the plexus and is by no means a complete description of the plexus. The following description will tend to make more clear the formation and position of the plexus.

The anterior primary divisions of the lower four cervical nerves, after passing dorsally to the vertebral artery and between the anterior and posterior parts of the intertransverse muscles, pass into the posterior triangle of the neck between the adjacent borders of the anterior and middle scalene muscles, where those of the fifth and sixth nerves receive a gray ramus communicans each from the middle cervical sympathetic ganglion, and those of the seventh and eighth nerves each receives a gray ramus from the inferior cervical sympathetic ganglion. The anterior primary division of the first thoracic is connected by two rami communicantes with the first thoracic sympathetic ganglion, and it divides into a smaller and a larger branch. The small branch passes along the intercostal space, as the first intercostal nerve and the large branch, after being joined by a twig from the second thoracic nerve, passes upward and laterally in front of the neck of the first rib and behind the apex of the pleural sac, into the lower part of the posterior triangle of the neck where it takes the formation of a plexus.

The trunks and branches are given off in the following manner: the infraclavicular part of the brachial plexus breaks up into its long branches in the lower part of the axilla; the long branches go exclusively into the arm.

The axillary portion of the brachial plexus is bounded medially by the serratus anterior, in front by the pectoral muscles and behind by the latissimus dorsi and the subscapularis muscles, between which it lies in a groove. Its constituents then lie in three cords in direct contact with the axillary artery in the axilla as shown with the arm in a horizontal position.

The position of the nerves of the brachial plexus in the axillary fossa and in the arm with relation to the axillary artery and nerve is outlined below.

[1] The median nerve will be described with the medial cord.

Position in the Axillary Fossa

1. The ulnar nerve lies between the axillary artery and vein.
2. The median nerve goes through the lower part of the fossa and is lateral to the axillary artery.
3. The radial nerve is posterior to the axillary artery and vein.
4. The musculocutaneous nerve is lateral to the axillary artery.

Position in the Arm

1. The ulnar nerve is medial to the brachial artery.
2. The medial nerve is also medial to the brachial artery.
3. The radial nerve is posterior to the brachial artery.

Muscles Supplied by the Nerves of the Brachial Plexus in Arm, Forearm and Hand.—*From the Lateral Cord:* the musculocutaneous nerve branches off, lies lateral to the axillary artery, and innervates three muscles of the arm: (1) the coracobrachialis; (2) the biceps; (3) the brachialis.

From the Medial Cord: the ulnar nerve branches off, lies between the axillary artery and vein in the axillary fossa; in the arm it is medial to the brachial artery, then passes posteriorly to pierce the medial intramuscular septum, and continues between the olecranon process and medial condyle of the humerus to supply only the muscles of the forearm and hand as listed below.

Muscles of the Forearm which the Ulnar Supplies

1. Flexor carpi ulnaris.
2. Flexor digitorum profundus (also supplied by the median nerve).

Muscles of the Hand which the Ulnar Supplies

1. Adductor pollicis.
2. Flexor pollicis brevis (supplied by the median also).
3. Volar and dorsal interossei.
4. Medial two lumbricals.
5. Muscles of the hypothenar eminence (intrinsic muscles of the little finger).

From the medial and lateral cord the median nerve also branches off, passes through the lower part of the axillary fossa to the arm where no muscles are supplied, to the forearm, and to the hand supplying muscles to the latter two parts. In the upper arm it lies medial to the brachial artery.

Muscles of the forearm supplied by the median nerve	1. The pronator teres
	2. The flexor carpi radialis
	3. The palmaris longus
	4. The flexor digitorum sublimus
	5. The flexor digitorum profundus
	6. The flexor pollicis longus
	7. The pronator quadratus

The last three are supplied by the volar interosseus branch of the median nerve.

Muscles of the hand supplied by the median nerve	1. The abductor pollicis brevis
	2. The flexor pollicis brevis (also ulnar nerve)
	3. The opponens
	4 The lateral two lumbricals

From the Posterior Cord: (*a*) The axillary nerve branches off, passes through the quadrilateral space, and supplies two muscles: (1) the deltoid; (2) the teres minor.

(*b*) The radial nerve also branches off this cord, lies posterior to the axillary artery in the axilla, and posterior to the brachial artery in the arm, following a course in the radial groove on the humerus to pierce the lateral intermuscular septum before entering the forearm. It supplies the muscles listed below.

Muscles of the arm supplied by the radial	1. The triceps
	2. The brachialis (also supplied by the musculocutaneous nerve)
	3. The anconeus
Muscles of the forearm supplied by the radial	1. Brachioradialis
	2. Extensor carpi radialis longus

Though branches of the radial nerve are cutaneous, muscular, articular, and terminal, only the terminal branches are considered here. The terminal branches of the radial nerve are (1) the deep radial (a motor branch), and (2) the superficial radial (a cutaneous nerve).

Muscles of the forearm supplied by the deep radial nerve	1. The extensor carpi radialis brevis
	2. The extensor digiti communis
	3. The extensor digiti quinti propius
	4. The extensor carpi ulnaris
	5. The supinator brevis
	6. The abductor pollicis longus
	7. The extensor pollicis longus
	8. The extensor pollicis brevis
	9. The extensor indicis propius

Causes, Signs and Symptoms of Brachial Plexus Paralysis.—Among infants paralysis sometimes results from violent manipulations of the body during birth; that involving the upper part of the lateral cord is one of the most common. Rending of the fifth cervical nerve and others going to the axillary and median nerves may give a partial or total loss of elevation and abduction at the shoulder and loss of flexion of the elbow, known as upper radicular brachial paralysis, or Erb's palsy. Paralysis of the muscles supplied by the medial cord is known as Klumpke's palsy.

The ulnar nerve passes so superficially over the elbow and back of the medial condyle that it is subject to blows, giving the condyle the name of "funny" bone. Damage here to the ulnar nerve, and possibly an open elbow joint, may result from injury to the epiphysis of the medial epicondyle, an injury which occurs more often prior to the eighteenth year when the epiphyseal line is still cartilaginous.

Because of the frequency of wounds on the front of the wrist and in the palm, producing paralysis, the following are some of the important locations of volar nerves which should be kept in mind.

The median nerve passes into the hand at a mid-point in front of the wrist. The volar branch of the ulnar nerve is superficial between the tendons of the flexor carpi ulnaris and the superficial flexor of the fourth digit. The main volar trunks of both ulnar and median break up beneath the center of the palmar aponeurosis, and branches of the ulnar course in the hypothenar eminence, on the way to the fourth and fifth digits. The characteristic wrist drop is due to paralysis of the deep radial nerve.

Paralysis of Muscles Supplied by Nerves of the Lateral Cord.—*The Musculocutaneous Nerve.*—Paralysis of the musculocutaneous nerve is rarely seen except in the cases of paralysis of the new-born. There results decreased power of flexion of the forearm, owing to complete paralysis of the biceps and partial paralysis of the brachialis. The sensation is impaired over the lateral aspect of the forearm, both back and front.

Paralysis of Muscles Supplied by Nerves of the Medial Cord.—*The Ulnar Nerve.*—Paralysis of the ulnar nerve may be caused frequently by incisor wounds on the forearm and wrist and also by fractures involving the medial condyle of the humerus. At the wrist the power of flexion is diminished and that of ulnar abduction is lost. In the hand the power of grasp is lessened in ring and little fingers. The interosseus muscles being out, there is difficulty in spreading the fingers. The hypothenar eminence disappears and the thenar eminence shows atrophy. The thumb cannot be adducted. Flexion deformity causes a "claw hand" due to paralysis of the lumbricals and interossei; there is overextension of the first phalanx and flexion of the second and the third phalanx, chiefly in the fourth and fifth fingers. Sensation will be lessened over the total area supplied by the nerve. As the interossei require a year for recovery, healing is slow and not always possible.

The Median Nerve (*Medial Cord*).—Paralysis of the median nerve usually accompanies other nerve injuries and may be due to fractures and deep lacerations.

In the forearm there is a loss of pronation; at the wrist, diminished flexion and a tendency toward ulnar abduction. In the hand the power of grasp is lessened (especially in the thumb and in the index finger). The fist cannot be clenched because of the loss of flexion of fingers, the thumb remains extended, adducted and applied to the index finger (Duchenne's ape hand), and the thumb cannot oppose any of the other fingers.

Sensation is lost over the palmar aspect of the thumb and lateral two and one-half fingers and over the distal ends of the same fingers to a varying degree. If the nerve is injured at the wrist, flexion of the wrist and fingers has less interference.

The prognosis is better than the ulnar, but not especially good for rapid recovery.

Paralysis of Muscles Supplied by the Nerves of the Posterior Cord.—*The Axillary Nerve.*—Paralysis of the axillary nerve may be caused by dislocation of the shoulder, by fracture of the surgical neck of the humerus, and by birth injuries.

There is a loss of normal contour of the shoulder and a subluxation of the shoulder joint. The arm is adducted close to the body because of inability to raise the arm. The arm is medially rotated, with the back of the hand turned forward.

The Radial Nerve (*Musculospiral*).—Paralysis of the radial, or musculospiral, nerve must frequently be distinguished from partial paralysis which involves the deep radial branch alone. The characteristic "wrist drop" is due to paralysis of the deep radial branch of the radial nerve. In a complete radial paralysis, the arm is flexed, pronated and the thumb is adducted.

Some of the causes which may produce a radial nerve paralysis are these:

1. Lead poisoning.
2. Use of crutches.
3. Fracture of the middle one-third of the humerus.

4. Pressure paralysis originating during operations.
5. A violent contraction of the triceps.
6. Any severe injury involving the middle one-third of the humerus because of the path of the radial nerve in the radial groove in this area.

Signs of paralysis of the radial nerve in the forearm include flexion of the arm, extension being impossible and pronation or supination is possible only by the biceps, which acts now most strongly on a flexed elbow joint.

In radial paralysis the wrist drops because of the loss of extension, as the deep radial is rendered useless. However, there may be a deep radial paralysis, although the main nerve is left intact.

In the hand the thumb is flexed and adducted. Some slight power of extension of the second and third phalanges of the fingers remains by means of the lumbricals and interossei.

Sensation is impaired over the posterior and lateral aspect of the forearm and lost to a varying extent over the distribution of the radial on the back of the hand.

The Deep Radial Nerve.—If the injury is in the forearm, the triceps muscle is not involved, and the deep radial nerve is alone involved in the paralysis. When the deep radial nerve is involved, the signs are the same as with a radial nerve involvement with the following exceptions:

In the forearm there is no loss of extension at the elbow and loss of supination is less, as the brachioradialis is left intact.

At the wrist there is a "wrist drop" but loss of extension is not as great because the extensor carpi radialis longus escapes. However, the patient shows a marked inability to extend the fingers.

Tests for Nerve Injuries of the Upper Extremity.—With exception of the upper arm type of brachial paralysis, an inspection of the fingers will reveal nerve involvement, even though the arm may be in a cast.

Isolated injuries to the musculocutaneous and axillary nerves are rare. With the upper type of brachial plexus lesion excepted, injuries to the axillary and musculocutaneous always involve either the median, ulnar, or radial nerves.

Any injury to the radial nerve, even to the lowest portion (the posterior interosseus branch), will result in loss of extension of the thumb; therefore, inability to extend the thumb completely immediately suggests a radial involvement.

In median nerve involvement injury in any location will affect the opponens pollicis, making it impossible to oppose the palmar surface of the thumb to the pads at the extremity of the fingers.

Whereas it may be possible to flex the terminal phalanx of the thumb through the long extensors, or the first phalanx by the action of the flexor pollicis brevis (which is partially supplied by the ulnar), it is impossible to rotate the thumb over the palm.

In injuries to the ulnar nerve the interosseus muscles are conspicuously involved and prevent the lateral movement of the fingers. This is revealed by inability to make a four finger cone.

Summary.—(1) Normal ulnar nerve permits a four finger cone. (2) Normal median nerve permits a five finger cone. (3) Normal radial nerve permits abduction and extension of the thumb. Therefore, it can be seen readily that the test of making a five finger cone and extension of the thumb reveals ulnar, median, and radial injuries.

Further confirmation may be made.

1. Radial injuries may be further confirmed by the presence of anesthesia over the dorsal surface of the base of the thumb, and also by the inability to elevate the wrist and extend the fingers at the metacarpophalangeal joints.
2. If the patient can make a four finger cone, but cannot oppose the thumb to it, he has a median nerve paralysis, showing also loss of sensation of the palmar surface of the first three fingers and inability to flex the index finger when the other fingers are extended.
3. If the patient cannot make a four finger cone, the ulnar nerve is involved as confirmed by the loss of sensation in the little finger and loss of lateral movement of the fingers also.

Chart for Muscles of Brachial Plexus

Lateral Cord

Musculocutaneous nerve supplies the following muscles:

Muscle	*Action*	*Origin*	*Insertion*
Brachialis	Flexion of forearm	Anterior border, ventral lower ⅜ of humerus	Coronoid process of ulna
Biceps (long head)	Supination and flexion of forearm	Supraglenoid tuberosity of scapula	Bicipital tuberosity of radius
Biceps (short head)	Same	Coracoid process of scapula	Same
Coracobrachialis	Forward flexion of arm	Coracoid process of scapula	Middle ⅓ shaft of humerus

Medial Cord

Ulna nerve supplies the following muscles in the forearm:

Flexor carpi ulnaris	Flexes and ulnar abducts the hand	Medial epicondyle of humerus	Pisiform bone, palmar aponeurosis base of 4th and 5th metacarpal
Flexor digitorum profundus	Flexes 3d phalanges, curls fingers	Briefly, the anterior surface of ulna	Bases of 3d row of phalanges

CHART FOR MUSCLES OF BRACHIAL PLEXUS (*Continued*)

MEDIAL CORD (*Contined*)

Ulna nerve supplies the following muscles in the hand:

Muscle	*Action*	*Origin*	*Insertion*
Flexor pollicis brevis	Flexes thumb at the base	Carpal ligaments, greater multangular	Base of 1st phalanx of thumb
Adductor pollicis	Helps adduct the thumb	Capitate, and 2d, 3d metacarpals	Base of 1st phalanx of thumb (ulnar side)
Volar interossei	Adducts toward mid-line	1st from ulnar side of own metacarpal. 2d. and 3d from radial sides of 4th and 5th metacarpals	1st and 2d into ulnar side base of 1st phalanx of same-digits. 3d and 4th in the radial side of 4th and 5th digits
Dorsal interossei	Abducts away from midline	Each of the four by two heads from adjacent sides of metacarpal bones	1st radial side index finger. 2d radial side 3d finger. 3d and 4th ulnar side of 3d and 4th fingers
Medial two lumbricals	Flexes the basal phalanges on the metacarpal bones and extends the terminal and middle phalanges	The lumbricals extend from the deep flexor tendons of the hand (palmar)	Are attached by small tendons to the radial side of the extensor tendon
Intrinsic muscles of the little finger; abductor digiti quinti, flexor digiti quinti brevis, opponens digiti quinti	Abducts 5th finger; flexes 1st phalanx, extends 2d and 3d phalanges		

Median nerve supplies the following muscles:

In the Forearm

Muscle	*Action*	*Origin*	*Insertion*
Pronator teres	Pronates the forearm	Medial epicondyle of the humerus and coronoid process of ulna	Lateral surface middle ⅓ of radius
Flexor carpi radialis	Flexes hand at wrist	Medial epicondyle of humerus	Base of 2d and 3d. metacarpal
Palmaris longus	Flexes hand at wrist	Medial epicondyle of humerus	Palmar aponeurosis
Flexor digitorum sublimis	Flexes 2d phalanges on 1st row of fingers	Medial epicondyle of humorus	Volar surface from 2d row phalanges

(The tendon of this muscle splits to let the tendon of the flexor digitorum profundus through)

Muscle	*Action*	*Origin*	*Insertion*
Flexor digitorum profundus	Flexes 3d phalanx on 2d and 2d on 1st	Anterior surface of ulna	Bases of 3d row phalanges
Flexor pollicis longus	Flexes distal phalanx of thumb	Anterior surface upper ⅔ radius	Base of distal phalanx thumb
Pronator quadratus	Pronates the forearm	Lower ¼ ulna volar surface	Lower ¼ volar surface radius

In the Hand

Muscle	*Action*	*Origin*	*Insertion*
Abductor pollicis brevis	Abducts the thumb	Greater multangular	Radial side at base 1st phalanx thumb
Flexor pollicis brevis	Flexes 1st joint of thumb	Carpal ligament, greater multangular	Same as above
Opponens pollicis	Opposes thumb to the other fingers	Annular ligament	Radial side 1st metacarpal
Lateral two lumbricals	Separates fingers	Tendon of flexor digitorum profundus	Tendon of extensor digitorum communis

Posterior Cord

Axillary nerve (circumflex) supplies the following muscles:

In the Shoulder

Muscle	*Action*	*Origin*	*Insertion*
Deltoid	Abduction of arm from the side to 90°	Outer $\frac{1}{3}$ of clavicle, acromium, lower border spine of scapula	Outer side, middle of humerus
Teres minor	Lateral rotation of arm	Upper $\frac{2}{3}$ axillary border scapula	Great tubercle of humerus

Radial nerve (musculospiral) supplies the following muscles:

In the Arm

Muscle	*Action*	*Origin*	*Insertion*
Triceps	Extension of forearm on the arm	Infraglenoid, tubercle of scapula; also above and below radial groove on posterior aspect of humerus	Olecranon process of ulna
Anconeus	Same as above	Lateral epicondyle	Same as above
Brachialis	Flexion of forearm on the arm	Lower $\frac{1}{2}$ shaft o humerus	Coronoid process of ulna

The radial nerve supplies the following muscles:

In the Forearm

Muscle	*Action*	*Origin*	*Insertion*
Brachioradalis	Supinates extended arm, pronates flexed arm, aids in flexing forearm	Supracondylar ridge of humerus	Styloid process of radius
Extensor carpi radialis longus	Same	Same	Base of 2d metacarpal dorsally

Deep radial supplies the following muscles:

In the Forearm

Muscle	*Action*	*Origin*	*Insertion*
Extensor carpi radialis brevis	Extends the hand	Lateral epicondyle	Bases 2d, 3d metacarpals
Extensor digitorum communis	Extends hand and phalanges of fingers (2d tn 5th)	Same	By four tendons middle and distal phalanges 2d to 5th fingers
Extensor digiti quinti proprius	Same as above	Same	Into the back of the fingers with the common extensor
Extensor carpi ulnaris	Extends hand and abducts it to radial side	Same	Back of the base of the 5th metacarpal
Supinator (brevis)	Supinates forearm	Same	Volar surface radius
Abductor pollicis longus	Abducts 1st metacarpal	Lateral margin dorsa surface of ulna	Base of 1st metacarpal radial side
Extensor pollicis longus	Extends 2d phalanx on 1st of thumb, helps radial abduction of hand	Dorsal middle $\frac{1}{3}$ radius	Base 2d phalanx of thumb
Extensor pollicis brevis	Extends thumb at metacarpo-phalangeal joint and abducts 1st metacarpal	Distal, dorsal $\frac{1}{3}$ of radius	Base of proximal phalanx of thumb
Extensor indicis proprius	Extends 1st phalanx on metacarpal and adducts the index finger, but mainly extends it	Dorsal aspect of the shaft of ulna	Deep aponeurosis of index finger

THE LUMBOSACRAL PLEXUS OF THE LOWER EXTREMITY

Formation of the Plexuses of the Lower Extremity.—The lumbosacral plexus is formed by the union of the anterior primary divisions of the lumbar, sacral, and coccygeal nerves. In about 50 per cent of the cases it receives a branch from the twelfth thoracic nerve. Its components are distributed to the lower extremity in a manner homogeneous to the distribution of the parts of the brachial plexus to the upper extremity.

The lumbar nerves are distributed in a manner similar to the nerves formed by the anterior (medial and lateral) cords of the brachial plexus and the sacral nerves are distributed in a manner similar to the distribution of the nerves from the posterior cord of the brachial plexus.

Partly for convenience of description and partly on account of the differences in position and course of some of the nerves arising from it, the lumbosacral plexus is subdivided into four parts: (1) the lumbar plexus; (2) the sacral plexus; (3) the pudendal plexus; (4) the coccygeal plexus.

It so happens that these plexuses overlap so that there is no definite line of demarcation between them in origin and distribution. However, they will be considered separately. Only the lumbar and the sacral will be reviewed here as incidental to the study of the nerves innervating the chief muscles of action of the lower extremity.

The Lumbar Nerves.—The anterior primary divisions of the five lumbar nerves increase in size from the first to the last. Each lumbar nerve is connected by one or two long slender rami with a lumbar sympathetic ganglion, the rami to the last two nerves being smaller. The first three nerves and the greater part of the fourth enter into the formation of the lumbar plexus, and the smaller parts of the fourth and fifth nerves commonly unite to form the lumbosacral trunk which takes part in the formation of the sacral plexus.

The Lumbar Plexus.—Although the lumbar plexus is ordinarily formed by the anterior primary divisions of the first three lumbar nerves and a part of the fourth, yet it is subject to considerable variation in the manner of its formation. It lies in the posterior part of the psoas muscle, in front of the transverse processes of the lumbar vertebræ and the medial border or the quadratus lumborum; its terminal branches are distributed to the lower part of the abdominal wall, the front and medial part of the thigh, the external genital organs, the front of the knee, the medial side of the leg, and the medial side of the foot.

The first and second lumbar nerves give collateral muscular branches to the quadratus lumborum; the second and third give similar branches to the psoas. The remaining branches are terminal branches.

The remaining nerves divide into anterior or ventral and posterior or dorsal divisions. The anterior divisions form a portion of the genito-femoral (genito-crural) nerve and the obturator nerve; the posterior division enters the lateral (external) cutaneous and the femoral (anterior crural) nerves.

All terminal branches of the plexus are formed in the substance of the psoas muscle; four of them, the iliohypogastric, the ilio-inguinal, the lateral (external) cutaneous, and the femoral (anterior crural), leave the muscle at its lateral border. The genito-femoral (genito-crural) passes through its anterior surface, and the obturator nerve passes through its medial border.

The Sacral Nerves.—The anterior primary divisions of the upper four sacral nerves enter the pelvis through the anterior sacral foramina and diminish in size progressively from above downward. The first sacral is the largest of the spinal nerves, the second is slightly smaller than the first, and the third and fourth are relatively still smaller. The fifth sacral, the smallest, enters the pelvis between the sacrum and the coccyx.

The anterior division of these nerves enters into the formation of three parts of the lumbosacral plexus: the sacral, pudendal, and the coccygeal parts, respectively.

The ordinary type of sacral plexus is commonly formed by the smaller part of the anterior divisions of the fourth lumbar nerve and the entire anterior division of the fifth lumbar nerve, together with the first and parts of the second and third sacral nerves.

The plexus lies in the pelvis on the anterior surface of the piriformis muscle and behind the pelvic fascia. It is also dorsal to the coils of the intestine, the sigmoid colon lying in front of the left plexus and the lower part of the ilium in front of the right plexus.

Muscular branches of the sacral plexus are as follows:

1. One or two small branches go to the piriformis muscle.

2. Posterior branches from the fourth and fifth lumbar, first sacral form the superior gluteal nerve as it passes out through the great sciatic foramen which, as it enters the buttocks, divides into two nerves, an upper which enters the gluteus medius, and a lower branch which supplies both the gluteus medius and the gluteus minimus and comes to an end in the tensor fasciæ latæ muscle.

3. The inferior gluteal nerve is formed from the fifth lumbar and the first and second sacral nerves. It ends in the gluteus maximus muscle.

4. "The nerve to the quadratus femoris" supplies the quadratus femoris and is formed by the fourth and fifth lumbar and the first and second sacral. This nerve also supplies the inferior gemellus muscle.

5. "Nerve of the obturator internus," formed from the fifth lumbar and first and second sacral, supplies the obturator internus and gives a branch to the superior gemellus.

6. The sciatic nerve. This nerve is the longest nerve not only of the sacral plexus but also of the whole body. It supplies the posterior part of the thigh and divides in the popliteal space. (Although this nerve is referred to as one trunk, it is in reality the lateral popliteal [peroneal] and the medial popliteal [tibial] which have one common sheath extending as far as the upper end of the popliteal space.) In the popliteal space it divides into the tibial and the common peroneal. The latter extends downward and forward to the upper part of the soleus muscle turning about the neck of the fibula to go forward to supply the anterior aspect of the leg, then breaking up into three branches: (1) the recurrent articular; (2) the superficial peroneal; (3) the deep peroneal. The tibial portion or branch of the sciatic nerve descends through the posterior aspect of the leg to a point between the medial malleolus and the tubercle of the calcaneus where it divides into terminal branches, the lateral plantar nerve and the medial plantar nerve, to supply the muscles of the plantar surface of the foot.

Muscles Supplied by the Nerves of the Lumbosacral Plexus.—The femoral (anterior crural) supplies:

1. The iliopsoas
2. The sartorius
3. The pectineus
4. The quadriceps femoris (rectus femoris, vastus internus, vastus externus and vastus intermedius)

The obturator nerve supplies:

1. The adductor longus
2. The adductor brevis
3. The gracilis
4. The obturator externus
5. The adductor magnus (also supplied by the sciatic nerve)

The superior gluteal nerve supplies:

1. The gluteus medius
2. The gluteus minimus
3. The tensor fasciæ latæ

The inferior gluteal nerve supplies:

1. The gluteus maximus

The sciatic nerve supplies:

1. The semitendinosus
2. The semimembranosus
3. The biceps (long head)
4. The adductor magnus (also supplied by the obturator)
5. The short head of the biceps is supplied by the peroneal portion of the sciatic nerve

The tibial nerve supplies:

1. The plantaris
2. The popliteus
3. The flexor digitorum longus
4. The flexor hallucis longus
5. The gastrocnemius
6. The soleus

The posterior tibial nerve supplies:

1. The tibialis posterior

The nerve to the quadratus femoris supplies:

1. The quadratus femoris muscle
2. The inferior gemellus

The nerve to the obturator internus supplies:

1. The obturator internus
2. The superior gemellus

The deep peroneal nerve supplies:

1. The extensor hallucis longus
2. The extensor digitorum longus
3. The extensor digitorum brevis
4. The tibialis anterior
5. The peroneus tertius

The superficial peroneal nerve supplies:

1. The peroneus longus
2. The peroneus brevis

Clinical Aspects of Nerves of the Lower Extremity.—In paralysis of the nerves of the lower extremity, consideration should be had from the viewpoint of surgical anatomy of the results of paralysis of the nerve chiefly affected, as of the great sciatic and its branches. With a paralysis of the sciatic the limb hangs flail-like, much in the position of one affected with advanced infantile paralysis. In addition to the results of paralysis of its two divisions, flexion at the knee will be lost, because of paralysis of the flexor muscles.

Paralysis of the peroneal (external popliteal) nerve: the extensors and peronei being paralyzed, the foot drops; it cannot be dorsiflexed at the ankle nor abducted at the mediotarsal joint. Adduction at the latter joint is impaired because of paralysis of the tibialis anterior. The arch of the foot is largely lost because of paralysis of the peroneus longus. Slight extension of the two distal phalanges of the four lateral toes is still possible by means of the interossei. Sensation is impaired over the distribution of the medial sural cutaneous and the deep and superficial peroneal nerves. With paralysis of the tibial (internal popliteal) nerve, the calf muscles, the flexors, and the muscles of the sole of the foot are paralyzed. The ankle cannot be plantar flexed.

Tests for Paralysis of the Nerves of the Lower Extremity.—Injuries to the femoral (anterior crural) nerve with loss of extension are rare.

Injuries to the sciatic and its two terminal divisions (tibial and peroneal) can be detected by inspection of the following movements: (1) If the toes can be extended, the peroneal portion of the nerve has escaped injury. (2) If the toes can be flexed, the tibial nerve has escaped. (3) If patient cannot extend the toes, there is peroneal involvement which is confirmed by loss of sensation in the cleft between the great and second toe, as well as by loss of dorsal flexion of the foot. (4) The inability to flex the toes means injury to the tibial which is confirmed by loss of sensation in the sole of the foot and inability to plantar flex the foot.

GENERAL SUMMARY OF METHODS OF TESTING FOR NERVE INJURIES OF UPPER AND LOWER EXTREMITIES

UPPER EXTREMITY

Musculospiral (*Radial*)

1. Inability to extend the thumb.
2. Inability to elevate wrist and extend fingers at the metacarpophalangeal joint.
3. Anesthesia over dorsal surface of base of thumb.

Median

1. Inability to rotate thumb over palm.
2. Inability to make a five finger cone.
3. Inability to flex index finger when others are extended or in hand clasping.
4. Inability to abduct thumb at right angle (because of shortening of adductor).
5. Anesthesia over palmar surface of first three fingers.

Ulnar

1. Inability to make a four finger cone.
2. Lack of lateral motion of fingers.
3. Anesthesia of little finger.

If the patient is able to make a five finger cone, both ulna and median nerve involvement may be eliminated.

LOWER EXTREMITY

Peroneal Nerve and Peroneal Portion of Sciatic (*External Popliteal*)

1. Inability to extend toes.
2. Inability to dorsal flex foot.
3. Anesthesia in cleft between great and second toes.

Tibial Nerve (*Internal Popliteal*) *and Tibial Portion of Sciatic*

1. Inability to flex toes.
2. Inability to plantar flex foot.
3. Anesthesia of sole of foot and toes.

CHAPTER VI

PHYSIOLOGY OF THERAPEUTIC EXERCISE

RELAXATION THEORY; MUSCLE REST

Introduction.—There are numerous indications for the use of exercise for therapeutics, but the value of the employment of rest and relaxation as a therapeutic measure has not been sufficiently recognized by the medical profession. It has been scientifically investigated and recorded that when mechanical work is done by a muscle, there are three phases: a latent period, a contraction period, and a relaxation period.

It is fitting, therefore, to take into consideration the value which may be obtained from the administration of therapeutic exercise with the thought in mind of the need of the muscle (and of the person as a whole) for relaxation between periods of use. A too vigorous and enthusiastic approach may result in a serious state, aptly termed a "residual neuromuscular hypertension." In brief, the exercise must be given with a fine discrimination of the condition of the patient, the results desired, and the expediency of the particular set of exercises to the need of the particular condition to be treated.

It is well known that for optimal muscular efficiency, a steady rate of activity is required at which muscular effort and muscular recovery may keep pace with each other. Oxidation apparently takes place in the relaxation phase only. In the absence of this phase of oxidation (during the recovery period), acid accumulates in the muscle and fatigue occurs. If regular stimulation of a muscle is continued after the contractions have reached their maximum amplitude, the irritability of the muscle becomes depressed, the contractions diminish in height, and ultimately the muscle fails to respond. The higher the rate of stimulation, the more rapid the onset and development of fatigue. Heat is produced during each of the three phases of muscular work and accelerates each phase of muscular contraction. Cold has the opposite effect.

In the best interest of administering therapeutic exercises, it is our opinion that an appreciation of the beneficial effects of rest and relaxation should be of prime importance, and a necessary adjunct to the scholastic background of those applying its principles.

Muscle Rest.—For a clear understanding of what constitutes muscle rest it is expedient to establish the "zero position." This is an intermediate position in which the prime mover and its particular antagonist are each exerting an equal force necessary to maintain the segment over which they have control at a neutral position. The intermediate position, which is that of rest or equilibrium, is not a state of inaction, but is an active state in which the opponents are evenly balanced—a state in which one may assume each to be exerting a pressure of 45 pounds. If both opposing muscle groups are paralyzed, the position of rest is the normal position of equilibrium between the two groups; however, a muscle weakened or paralyzed, whether from injury of muscle, nerve, or central cell, is rested when its opponent is in a state of relaxation and elongation beyond the state normally necessary to produce a condition of equilibrium with its opponent. In this way a weakened muscle is prevented from being stretched and irritated by the contraction of its opponent. Since rest is the basic treatment of inflammation, then only by the "zero" position can the door be closed on all sources of irritation, and cord, nerve, "receptive substance" and muscle be at physiological rest.

It is from this position that after-gains in function are to be sought. The next question is the recognition of the minimum, so that the muscle may ultimately be coaxed up to the maximum—the ideal aim of treatment. Treatments are begun at "zero." Although the amount of work at this minimum is slight, it must be remembered that it really represents the maximum function of the muscle for the time being, and as such may soon become exhausted. In the same way normal individuals soon tire if asked to continue an action for some time and to the full extent.

Rest as an Active State.—When a muscle contracts in response to stimulation and produces motion of a segment of the body, the action is spoken of as "kinetic" or "phasic." Moreover, if the muscles remain contracted merely to hold a body segment stationary, the contraction is called "postural" or "static." Even though a muscle is not contracting to produce motion, it may still be in a state of muscular activity or in a postural or static state. Ordinarily when kinetic motion occurs, the number of stimuli reaching a muscle fiber from an anterior horn cell may be between five and twenty-five per second. If stimuli become intense, the number may reach ninety per second. "Residual muscular hypertension" is apparently synonymous with a condition which has been called forth by pressure and results in anxiety, irritability, restlessness, and disturbance of emotions. For example, those who may have had to remain in one position for several hours and whose muscles are in a state of postural or static contraction during that time will be relieved by kinetic or phasic exercises. The same principle may be applied to a patient who for some reason (known perhaps only to himself) is under an emotional strain or pressure from some problem and is unconsciously maintaining his muscles in a "static" hypertension. To give this patient active exercise without first inducing a degree of relaxation is undesirable.

Rest as a Therapeutic Measure.—Although apparently there is little or no fatigue resulting from postural or tonic contractions, actually "tonic" contractions are fatiguing out of all proportion to the physiological changes taking place in the muscles or the rate of response in the nerve. Marked residual tension or "contraction reminder" may result from prolonged tonic contraction; thus, although static effort as compared with dynamic effort exercises but little influence on metabolism, the "static" type is the one which produces "hypertension" and fatigue.

In many conditions it is impossible to stress adequately the value of rest as a therapeutic measure. Therapeutic rest can be measured only by a conscious reaction in the individual patient and relies, therefore, on his own intelligence and behavior. He must be taught *how* to rest and *how* to remain below the point of fatigue in and during the administration of therapeutic exercises. The same point carries through for the individual in ordinary life; one who has become accomplished in achieving relaxation often is capable of more work than one who cannot slow up at will. After periods of overwork the muscles tend to become tense and the brain overactive; under these circumstances it will take some time to be able to slow up and relax.

How to Induce Relaxation.—The patient should be given training in conscious relaxation or "progressive relaxation." It has been brought out by others that periods of intense activity should be followed by periods of conscious relaxation. If the patient is constantly fatigued and nervous, he must be guided in measures which will tend to protect him from undue stimuli, from both external forces and internal forces. Many times he must be taught how to sleep, how to control emotions, and how to adapt dietary knowledge to his needs, as well as how to relax; for without these measures all the doctrination of relaxation will become void.

APPLICATION OF FUNDAMENTAL MOVEMENTS USED IN THERAPEUTIC EXERCISE

Indication for the Employment of Therapeutic Exercise.—Properly administered, therapeutic exercise exerts a potent usefulness in the practice of medicine. Exercise should be given, as a rule, only after careful examination of the cardiovascular system and should be prescribed according to a definite plan. The technician administering the exercises should be equipped with a thorough knowledge of anatomy, kinesiology, and pathology in order to interpret more clearly the prescription for exercise given by the physician.

Exercise should be thought of not simply in terms of strengthening an individual muscle or group of muscles by constant and vigorous usage, but rather as an important aid in rehabilitating patients suffering from many widely varied systemic, as well as local bodily conditions. For example, in an attempt gradually to increase the heart's tolerance for exertion, the physician may prescribe carefully graded exercise for patients suffering from cardiac disease. Exercises, specific in nature, passive in type to increase the peripheral collateral circulation of a patient with a thrombo-angiitis obliterans, may be indicated. Although these exercises may affect the strength of the skeletal muscles, such is not the purpose of the prescription for the exercise. Conversely, a patient with a functional type of kyphosis is given a specific set of exercises for the express purpose of strengthening the skeletal muscles of the upper portion of the back, in order to bring about a corrected posture of that region.

Classification of Movements Used in the Administration of Therapeutic Exercise.—Exercise, which means "to set in motion," may be performed either by the patient alone or with assistance, and are classified broadly as active and passive types of exercise. In order to understand more clearly the learning of new movements, as in muscle re-education, the significance of the neuromuscular mechanism involved in the process must be clearly understood by a review of the phenomenon of musular control. As it has been stated earlier,[1] skeletal muscles are classified as to the rôle they assume in joint motion, as well as to activity as directed by the patient's will, or performed without his volition.

There are prime movers (protagonists or agonists), antagonists, those which act as synergists, and fixers.

Prime movers are the muscles which actually produce an intended movement. The antagonists are those which tend to oppose the action of the prime movers. The synergists so modify the action of the first two that the intended movement is performed smoothly, free from shocks or jolts, and with the least expenditure of energy. Without collaboration of these various groups the apparently simple acts of everyday life would of necessity be difficult and awkward.

[1] Chapter II, p. 14.

Still another motivating force which contributes smoothness and grace in the process of performing an active exercise is the doctrine of relaxation as has been mentioned. When a group of muscles contract normally, the respective antagonists are made to relax at the same time. Known as Sherrington's Law of Reciprocal Innervation, this is a positive and not a negative action.

Enunciation of the Law of Reciprocal Innervation.—Much debate concerning the possibility of the simultaneous contraction of antagonistic muscles or muscle groups led to extended research on this subject.

New light was eventually thrown on the subject by Sherrington's exhaustive work, the outcome of which was the enunciation of the law of reciprocal innervation, the substance of which is as follows: "When a decerebrate or spinal preparation executes a muscular movement, augmentation of contraction never proceeds concurrently in antagonistic muscles, and similarly diminution of contraction in antagonists does not occur concomitantly."[1] The conception is that as contraction progresses in a muscle, contra-active activity diminishes in the antagonist. Contraction may thus be present in two opposing muscles at the same time, but in a reciprocal relationship; for example, if one muscle contracts to nine-tenths of its maximum, the opposing muscle may be contracted to one-tenth of its fullest extent.

Classification of Activity According to the Neuromuscular Control.—Muscular activity falls into two main divisions, active and passive.

A. Active purposeful movement is prompted and executed under the direction of the will of the patient himself, and employs the three types of neurons. It involves the upper and lower neurons, the motor and sensory nerves, the myoneural junction and the muscle itself. This group is further subdivided into various minor groups. Neither passive movements nor muscular action initiated by an electrical impulse can as exclusively and favorably influence the neuromuscular arc as active movements. This intricate mechanism is so complete that when the command for movement is given by the brain cells there is always a clear mental picture of the intended movement. For a movement impulse to express itself, it must be controlled by the sensory nerves; for the will and the sensibility are functions inseparably connected with each other. Because of this intimate relationship between brain and muscle, voluntary purpose-

[1] Fulton, J. F.: Muscular Contraction and the Reflex Control of Movement, Baltimore, Williams & Wilkins Co., pp. 447, 1926.

ful movements are of vital importance in the therapeutics of restoring various nerve-muscle disturbances to normalcy; illustrative examples are flaccid and spastic paralysis, locomotor ataxia, and various other forms of muscular dystrophies and nerve disorders. The term neuromuscular re-education is applied to the particular technique employed for restoration of function.

The indications for this type of muscular activity are those in which motion is imparted to a joint segment by voluntary contraction and relaxation of the muscles controlling the movement of that segment. It is termed free when it is not aided by external forces and the patient makes the complete effort by himself without assistance from the operator and against gravity. It is used in general to procure muscular development and stimulation of the vital organs, to stimulate mentality, to re-educate and develop the neuromuscular apparatus (coördination), and to increase or maintain lost joint function.

This form of exercise can be further classified as positive (raising the arm sidewards); static (holding the position); and negative (lowering the arm slowly).

Some specific indications for active exercises are posture exercises, spinal curvatures, weak or potential flat feet, weak abdominal wall, muscular disturbances as poliomyelitis, spastic paralysis, cardiac disabilities, peripheral vascular disease, restoration of function following trauma, as well as functional and mental diseases. This type of exercise lends itself well to the field of occupational therapy in which the patient is taught to use his hands and legs in skills and crafts through the process of learning new activities.

1. Assistive movements, as the name implies, are useful in supplementing voluntary effort where normal muscle power is deficient. For example, the patient is requested to make an active effort to move the part while the operator or some mechanical agent assists in the movement, as in the re-education of a weak deltoid when the patient, in the supine position, is asked to bring the arm to a 90° abduction. Assistance is offered by the technician for the first and third parts of the movement while the patient alone performs during the second part. Indications for this type of exercise are chiefly in mobilization of joints in cases in which a muscle is being re-educated to assume full responsibility for its own activities and in assistive movements used to a great extent in the early treatment of poliomyelitis. This form of exercise calls for unusual judgment on the part of the operator, who should watch closely for signs of fatigue and fibrillation. This form of exercise also permits the feeble muscle to act by eliminating checks to action, counterbalancing the

weight of the limb, inducing relaxation of the opposing group, and eliminating friction, gravity, and inertia.

2. Resistive active movements are those in the course of which the technician resists the efforts of the patient, or the patient may use his own physiological antagonistic group of muscles to produce the resistance. The technician offers just as much resistance as the patient is able to overcome. These movements exert distinct advantages over purely active ones for the following reasons.

Groups of muscles may be isolated by eliminating the co-action of their antagonists, through the operation of relaxation by the law of proprioceptive innervation.

By the same token protective spasm may be lessened. For example, resistance to knee flexion relaxes the overactive quadriceps.

Contraction may be brought about very early in apparently totally paralyzed muscles. It has been shown that some patients can perform resistive movements sooner than they can the corresponding purely active ones in which the same muscles are called into action.

The work done by the patient can be graduated in any amount desired.

By virtue of the first two reasons, resistive exercise offers an excellent method of studying muscular action and relative strength.

Through muscular isolation, inflammations and joint pain resulting from pressure and interarticular friction may be lessened and hence a greater degree of motion is obtained.

Mechanical devices may be so arranged as to offer resistance to the action of a particular part. All resistive exercise should be guided by the principle that the strength of muscles is reduced in direct proportion to the state of contraction or its relative length. Therefore, the strength of resistance applied must be different for the different phases of the movement. Usually the least resistance is offered at the beginning and last one-third and the greatest resistance is offered at the middle one-third of the arc. The optimum power of the muscle is at the middle one-third of the arc.

Gravity may be used in offering resistance to the part to be moved, in which the use of the patient's own body weight is the factor of resistance; however, the vital importance of effecting relaxation when utilizing gravity for the performance of a movement must be fully realized. Occasionally when a movement is impeded by adaptive shortening of its antagonist, and attempted increase in movement is painless, stretching by the use of gravity may be used as a definite curative agent.

If the operator is supplying the resistance, he may perform a movement while the patient resists. This is termed an eccentric movement, during which the muscle actually lengthens. When the movement is done by the patient while the operator resists, the movement is a concentric one during which the muscle decreases its length or shortens. The amount of resistance given in a concentric resisted movement depends on the operator, whereas in eccentric active resistive movement the patient arranges the matter of resistance for himself. It is worthy to note here that when a muscle is recovering from a paralysis and is in an early stage, eccentric movements are to be avoided and concentric movement will be found of the utmost service during all the earlier stages of treatment.

The raising of the patient's arm in abduction is an active one if performed by the sole effort of the patient himself; it is a passive movement if applied by the operator to the patient without the latter offering either assistance or resistance.

B. The action of passive movements must not be confused with manipulation of a stiff joint to break adhesions or the stretching of shortened muscles. Neither should it be recognized as a synonym for the term "relaxing movements," since passive movements are in no way concerned with releasing tension of muscular tissue. Passive is a descriptive term meaning the opposite of active. In passive movements the sensory-association-motor neuron synapse is in no way involved, whereas this unit is definitely and vitally concerned in the phenomenon of relaxation.

The significance of passive movement will be more fully appreciated by noting its practical application in physical medicine.

1. Passive exercise may be used preliminary to active movement when the latter may retard progress of complete joint motion.

2. Passive exercise acts to improve the return lymph and blood circulation by virtue of compression and joint motion.

3. Passive movement helps retain full amplitude of joint motion by the prevention of contractures, the shortening of muscles, and the formation of adhesions.

4. Passive movement acts to maintain normal positional sense, as in knowing with the eyes closed when the arm is abducted shoulder high.

5. Passive movement serves to maintain nerve power by stimulation through stretching and shortening of muscles. It increases the suppleness of joints, maintains nerve power by joint pressure which involves the sensory motor impulses.

Whereas the patient does not participate actively in passive motion, there should be a mental awareness accompanying the process to differentiate this movement from manipulative procedures in which the patient does not participate actively or mentally.

C. In manipulative procedure, the operator's goal is to break adhesions or to mobilize a tightened contracture or stiff joint. In manipulation, the physician should designate the degree of force to be used as "painless movement" or "movement to the point of pain," or grade the movements by number according to severity, or range of motion to be achieved, as the maximum number of degrees of flexion or extension desired. It is believed that at all times the limit at which pain occurs is the point to discontinue further forced movement. Severe forced manipulations are at times carried out by the physician in charge, and should be, of necessity, an operative procedure where the patient is placed under an anesthetic to attain the maximum degree of relaxation of the muscles. However, this procedure is frowned upon by many physicians.

"Muscle Setting Exercises."—These exercises may be classified as intermittent contraction and relaxation of muscles without joint motion.

This rather unsatisfactory term, "muscle setting exercise," has been applied to a type of voluntary muscle contraction which does not involve joint motion. It is admirably adapted to conditions of fracture or joint injury to arm or leg. Though the patient's leg may be encased in a cast, still he is able to carry on muscular contractions, thus improving the circulation and the muscle tone.

Aids in Muscle Training.—In treating weak muscles by means of active exercise there is always a danger of overtaxing the optimum capacity for work which would hinder the progress of recovery. In order to minimize this danger, the technician finds it helpful to employ certain procedures to lessen the factors of gravity and friction. Though some of these will be mentioned here, they by no means cover the possibilities of aids.[1]

Postural Aids.—The aim is to place the body in a position favorable to the elimination of gravity to a greater or lesser extent. In treating a weak deltoid muscle the patient is placed on his back with the arm to the side resting on a smooth board covered with talcum powder, which reduces friction and readily enables the arm to be carried to a position of abduction. The use of roller skates on the foot may accomplish much the same effect with the lower extremity.

[1] A more detailed description is presented in Chapter III.

Sling Suspension.—Still another method for minimizing gravity is to suspend the extremity in a sling about six inches from the bed or table. Again in this position the leg may be abducted and adducted and the knee flexed with comparative ease and without straining the muscles involved. An elastic band may be attached to the lower end of the sling, which then offers opportunity for increased amplitude of motion, or it may be used as a resistance mechanism when that form of exercise is deemed advisable.

Underwater Exercise.—These movements are performed in a therapeutic pool or a tank constructed for home use. Exercise in a pool must not be confused with swimming. It is useful because the buoyancy of the water lessens gravity and makes possible the application of therapeutic exercise, which is especially important when the muscles have been badly damaged by disease, trauma, or atrophied from disuse.

Contraindications for the Use of Therapeutic Exercise.—As has been indicated, the uses for therapeutic exercise not only are varied and numerous, but also cover many of the fields of medicine, some of which are orthopedic, surgical, medical, psychiatric, as well as recreational and prophylactic.

As for the contraindication to this valuable adjunct to physical medicine, the greatest contraindication lies in the maladministration of, and not the prescription for, it in any given case. Therapeutic exercise is rarely contraindicated, for a definite amount of exercise is normal for all living, and motion for various parts of the body is essential to the maintenance of physiological processes. The great danger, therefore, lies in the choice of an exercise, the manner in which the exercises are being performed, the times at which they are given, and the duration for which they are to be used.

It is necessary to stress here again that it is better to administer the exercises in small, oft-repeated doses than to overdo them at any particular time at the risk of undesirable effects of fatigue.

Specific written instructions by the physician carried out by well-trained and experienced technicians are to be much desired to prevent the misuse of this valuable modality

CHAPTER VII

SPECIAL APPLICATIONS OF THERAPEUTIC EXERCISE

MANAGEMENT BY EXERCISE OF WEAK AND POTENTIAL FLAT FEET

THE pathomechanics of the foot will not be considered here, but if actual deformity is present, exercises sometimes may be prescribed for the patient; however, it is more often found necessary to place the limb in plaster after a thorough manipulation of all the joints of the foot. This procedure lies in the physician's hands, but later re-education exercises may be needed for complete restoration of function.

In all remedial exercises for pathological conditions of the feet the most important point to observe, if success is to be insured, is so to arrange the exercises that weight bearing may be assumed little by little and that each addition is so slight that the patient is unable to recognize any increase in strain imposed upon them.

It is essential that every precaution be taken to prevent lowering of the longitudinal arch of the foot when the patient is a bed case, especially over a long period of time. The weight of the blankets frequently induces a "drop foot" which will be retained after the illness. As a precaution every measure should be taken to maintain a good position of the feet during the period of illness. A cradle or footboard may be placed at the foot of the bed to support the bedding. Daily foot massage and exercises, or splinting the feet if the patient is too ill for treatment are recommended. No patient convalescing from a serious illness should ever be allowed to use his feet for their weight bearing function until muscular strength of the intrinsic muscles of the feet and of the long muscles which help support the arches have been restored.

It is well to note here also that when the patient is eventually placed in the weight bearing position preliminary to the giving of walking exercises, he should be shod with a pair of well broken-in shoes with good heels and not permitted to begin walking in bedroom slippers. The need for this precaution can be seen readily, as the ordinary type of bedroom slipper has no heel and does not protect the already weakened arches of the patient's feet.

Metatarsalgia.—This condition is a far more common cause of pain and disability than any other form of foot trouble. By far the most common cause of metatarsalgia is not, as thought frequently, traumatic neuritis, but rather traumatic arthritis, bursitis, periostitis, or a combination of all three. The main remedy is muscle-training, supplemented by various supports and pads for the long arch and the transverse arch, orthopedic shoes, and even elastic bands which encircle the arch. The patient's re-educational process is begun with passive exercises leading to active resistive exercises, first in a non-weight bearing position, then on his feet, at which time he is given balancing steps and foot placing exercises before actual walking is begun.

General Classification of Weak or Flat Feet.—Synonyms: Flat foot, pronated foot, pes planus, fallen arches.

Types of Weakened Feet:

1. A strained foot is the beginning of a weak foot, the result of abnormal functioning of the foot resulting in tiredness. Many cases have their beginning in ill fitting or pointed-toe shoes. In avoidance of pain, the weight is shifted to abnormal positions.

2. In a relaxed incipient weak foot the arch is depressed upon weight bearing but regains normal position when pressure is removed.

3. In a flattened weak foot the depressed arch does not regain its normal position when weight bearing is relieved.

4. A rigid weak foot is caused by muscular spasm.

5. A congenital flat foot (pes planus) exists from birth. It is characteristic of certain races, negroid, indian.

6. A traumatic foot because of injury changes to an abnormal position.

7. A paralyzed foot or flail foot is the abnormality following poliomyelitis.

Etiology of Weak Feet.—(1) Faulty alignment. Tibial torsion, knock knees, bow legs, rotation of thigh, or any condition which causes improper functioning of the foot, will tend to throw it in malposition either of abduction and pronation, or adduction and supination. (2) Faulty nutrition and long continuous weight bearing, finally causing loss of muscle tone with stretching of ligaments. (3) Faulty tarsal development. (4) Improper shoes and stockings. (5) Sudden changing from high to low heels. (6) Shortened calf muscles. (7) Hallux valgus, often resulting in bunions. (8) General weakness following acute infectious disease. (9) An inherent muscular weakness. (10) Disease of bones and joints. (11) Trauma. (12) Partial paralysis. (Typical of this type are residual weaknesses of the musculature of the foot post-poliomyelitis.) (13) Faulty postural attitudes. (14) Continuous weight bearing positions on hard surfaces, such as cement floors.

Treatment of Weak Feet.—The object of treatment is to regain normal motion by muscle re-education, to correct faulty attitudes by correct position of the feet while standing and walking, and to restore faulty foot structure. Adhesive strapping to support weakened muscles and ligaments, felt padding to support the arch, raising the inner border of soles and heels to correct pronation in certain cases. Contrast baths to the feet to improve circulation may be prescribed as supplements to proper exercise to stretch the calf muscles and to strengthen and shorten the anterior group. Support the feet with proper shoes, well fitted by competent sales person. The position of the feet while standing and walking is very important. They should be parallel in the weight bearing position always with the toes pointing slightly inward.

Flat Foot Exercises

Non-weight Bearing.

Lying on back, bend and abduct knees, bringing feet sole to sole.

Lying on back, hips flexed, with legs against wall, bring toes down as far as possible.

Lying on back, knees straight, with feet against wall, parallel and together, keep big toes and heels together and rotate thighs outward.

Sitting on chair, bring toes together and heels far apart. Raise forefoot off floor.

Sitting position, with soft rubber ball placed between feet, grasp ball with soles of feet and raise it from floor.

Sitting position with feet six inches apart and parallel. Pick up a marble with toes of left foot and place it behind the right heel.

Sitting position with knees semi-flexed, heels on the floor fifteen inches apart. On one, dorsi-flexion; two, extension; three, bring big toes together, heels far apart; and on four, back to position of dorsi-flexion.

Weight Bearing in Standing Position.

Bring left foot across and parallel to right foot, keeping foot one inch off floor. Hold this position for one minute. Reverse.

Stand on an elevated box, or step, with the edge of the step under the transverse arch, and with the toes extending over the edge. Bend, or curl, the toes over the edge of the step.

Stand with the toes turned in, heels apart; rise on toes, keeping the knees straight, throwing the weight on the outer borders of the feet.

Stand with feet parallel, rise to the outer border of the feet with the toes flexed and return to the first position without letting the arches sag.

Walk with the weight on the outer borders of the feet, keeping the feet parallel with the toes flexed.

General Rules to be Observed in Giving Foot Exercises.—At first use exercises with the patient in non-weight bearing positions only; later advance to the standing position.

Do not in any instance exercise a painful foot.

Avoid excessive heel raising and circumduction of the foot as an exercise.

Remember that well made and properly fitted shoes aid in the relief of many ailments of the feet.

When sitting, the patient should be advised to cross ankles, resting the feet on the outer borders. The long arch is then in a rest position, avoiding strain on weak arches. This position is avoided if the foot is supinated because of weak peroneal muscles.

When standing, he should keep the feet parallel, the weight of the body equally on both feet, with the quadriceps taut.

When walking, he should place the feet parallel, toes pointed straight forward, with the weight on the outer and forepart of the foot, two-thirds of weight on forepart of foot and one-third on heel.

Procedures Which May be Employed in Conjunction With Foot Exercises.—*Contrast Baths.*—Use two vessels, one with comfortably warm water, and the other with cold tap water. Place feet first in the warm water for four minutes, then in the cold water for one minute, alternately, for four or five times, ending with the warm water. (Avoid any temperature above warm if the patient is suffering from diabetes or arteriosclerosis.)

Massage.—Massage following the bath should be deep and rhythmical. Avoid massage over bony prominences, such as the shin bone and ankle bone. Begin at the lower end of the muscle and massage to the upper part: from the ankle to the knee, from the forepart of the foot to the ankle, and from the tips of the toes to the foot, to aid in emptying the parts of any old-standing edema.

MANAGEMENT BY EXERCISE OF WEAKNESSES OF THE ABDOMINAL WALL

General Anatomy and Action of Muscles of the Abdominal Wall and Related Muscles of the Back.—In the abdominal region the external layer is represented by the external oblique muscle; the middle layer by the internal oblique; and the inner layer by the transversalis, while the ventral part of the thoraco-abdominal wall is composed singly by the rectus abdominis muscles, one on each side and parallel with the mid-sagittal line.

The normal position of the spine largely depends on the tone of the abdominal muscles, and because the muscles of the abdominal wall must be considered as being essentially a part of the musculature of the anterior aspect of the joints of the back, those muscles of the back which are not classified with the shoulder girdle or shoulder joint will be considered here as well as the diaphragm, which, as an accessory muscle of respiration, is also the physiological antagonist of the abdominal muscles. The origins and insertions are given briefly here.

External Oblique

Origin: Fifth to twelfth ribs.

Insertion: Anterior one-third of iliac crest, anterior superior spine and abdominal aponeurosis.

Action: Compresses abdominal contents, flexes trunk anteriorly and laterally.

Internal Oblique

Origin: Outer one-third Poupart's ligament, anterior two-thirds iliac crest, lumbar fascia.

Insertion: Tenth to twelfth ribs, posterior; seventh to ninth ribs, anterior; linea alba, conjoined ligament into the pubic crest.

Action: Compresses abdominal contents, and flexes and rotates trunk.

Transversalis

Origin: Outer one-third Poupart's ligament, anterior two-thirds of iliac crest, deep surface of seventh to twelfth ribs, and transverse processes of lumbar vertebræ.

Insertion: Linea alba, conjoined tendon into the pubic crest.

Rectus Abdominis

Origin: Symphysis and crest of the pubis.

Insertion: Fifth, sixth and seventh ribs. (This muscle is believed to have its origin and insertions reversed by some authorities.)

Action: The action is to depress the thorax, and flex the spinal column. When the thorax is fixed, it helps to flex the pelvis upon the trunk.

Quadratus Lumborum

Origin: Anterior layer, transverse process fifth to second lumbar vertebræ. Posterior layer, internal iliac crest and iliolumbar ligament.

Insertion: Anterior layer, inferior border twelfth rib and body of twelfth thoracic vertebra. Posterior layer, inferior margin twelfth rib and transverse processes fourth to first lumbar ones.

Action: The action is chiefly lateral flexion of the spinal column, and when both act together they extend the spinal column.

The Erector Spinæ Group (Sacrospinalis group)

1. Iliocostalis.
2. Longissimus.
3. Spinalis.

Origin: Spines of the lumbar vertebræ, posterior surface of sacrum, crest of ilium and lumbar fascia.

Insertion: By progression upward into the spinous and transverse processes of the vertebræ, finally the ribs, occiput and mastoid process.

Action: They perform extension of the spine and are the means of holding the trunk erect.

The Diaphragm.—The diaphragm will be reviewed here because of its antagonistic action of the abdominal muscles. The diaphragm is not a muscle group acting directly on the lungs, but one which increases the capacity of the chest by compressing the abdominal organs like a piston. This is rendered possible by the reciprocal relaxation and elongation of the abdominal muscles.

Origin and Insertion: The diaphragm consists of a pair of muscles, which arise each from opposite sides of the thoracic wall and are inserted into a central tendon. It is a dome-shaped muscle which is attached to the lower margin of the thorax and to the upper lumbar vertebræ, and separates the thoracic and abdominal cavities

Action: It is believed by some to cause inspiration by enlarging the thoracic cavity. However, there is a discrepancy in theories concerning the action of this muscle, and it is thought to play a less important part in inspiration than is usually believed for it. It aids in defecation, parturition, and vomiting by the pressure it exerts on the abdominal viscera. It may also act to constrict the esophagus.

General action of all the muscles of the abdominal wall together cause constriction of the abdominal cavity.

The Importance of a Strong Abdominal Wall.—The most important muscles in the teaching of good body mechanics are the abdominal group. Equally true is their importance in the etiology of many medical diseases, especially in those cases which are complicated by a visceroptosis. Teaching the control of abdominal musculature and also the ability to use it in lying, sitting, and standing positions is the ultimate goal of this section.

1. Strong abdominal muscles act as a support for the best position of the chest and upper back.

2. The abdominal wall is the controlling factor in the tilt of the pelvis.

3. The abdominal wall is a mechancial support or foundation of the framework upon which the upper extremity rests.

4. When the abdomen is held up, there is a corresponding lift given to the chest.

5. There must be distinguished the difference between holding the abdomen "up" and "pulling" it in. The latter should be discouraged, because it interferes with normal breathing.

6. Strong abdominal muscles are important as a support of the abdominal organs, as a preventive of constipation, and as an aid to digestion. It is the major health measure in preventing and overcoming many organic ills.

7. A strong abdominal wall should supersede the use of supports and girdles.

Pathomechanics of Abdominal Muscles.—Under certain conditions, namely, paralysis of the back extensors, pathological conditions of the spine, pregnancy, and poor body mechanics due to habitual slump (purely functional), the line of gravity is displaced backward of the sacro-iliac joint, the balance of the body as a whole is maintained by accentuating the lumbar curve. In this position the abdominals are relaxed and stretched; consequently there is a ptosis of the abdominal wall. In this case the inclination of the pelvis backward is increased, the hip joint stands in a flexory position to the pelvis and the lumbar lordosis is often compensated for by a correspondingly strong dorsal kyphosis.

A great deal is said about the lordosed back and the evils which accompany it, but comparatively little is heard of the flat back. This condition is very difficult to distinguish except in the standing position, in which the sacrum is set in an abnormally vertical position, with the coccyx running forward well between the legs. This is in marked contrast to the lordosed position, where the sacrum is set in an unduly horizontal position, with the coccyx directed backwards. Though it may be thought that examination of the abdominal muscles has little to do with the examination of the back, this is an error, as the muscles of the abdominal wall must be considered as being essentially a part of the musculature of the anterior aspect of the joints of the back. As a flaccid abdominal wall almost invariably goes with a lordosed back, this combination produces what is commonly known as a ptosis posture. Everted feet, bent knees, bowed shoulders, and sunken chest go with it inevitably, and so produce the general condition that proves the adage that we grow old because we stoop, and do not stoop because we grow old. The flat back patient will stretch out both legs and flatten the back down against the bed in order to obtain rest. The patient with sacro-iliac trouble will keep the knee and hip of the affected side flexed; the patient with trouble in any of the lumbar joints will find this position intolerable unless both knees and hips are bent.

An important factor in overcoming the above pathomechanics is the strengthening of the abdominal wall by certain activities and exercises.

General Principles Guiding Abdominal Exercise.—Good judgment is imperative in the administration of abdominal exercises. The number of times they are done is guided by signs of fatigue, and the total number given. A few often repeated is a good criterion.

Abdominal exercises in general should begin with those requiring a supine position and progress to a more strenuous form in sitting and standing positions.

The combined strength of the muscles of the abdominal wall is much less than that of the diaphragm. If the airways are open, the increase of pressure of the abdominal muscles leads to narrowing of the lower aperture of the thoracic cavity and the diaphragm is forced further into the thoracic cage.

If the airways are closed, however, the compression of the abdominal muscles will fail to force the diaphragm upward, and concerted action of the diaphragm and abdominal muscles will produce an enormous increase in intra-abdominal pressure. Therefore, the most effective combination for expiration is contraction of muscles depressing and narrowing the thoracic cage combined with active contraction of the muscles of the abdominal wall and relaxation of the diaphragm. It is urgent that the patient should be cautioned against closing the air passages while taking abdominal exercises because the intra-abdominal pressure is increased and may produce untoward effects as in postherniorrhaphy and other postoperative conditions where pressure downward on the abdominal contents is undesirable.

In the presence of lordosis, hip flexion is contraindicated, because it involves the use of the hip and trunk flexor muscles, the iliopsoas. These most likely have already been shortened by position and further strengthening would increase the lordosis. An example of exercise misapplied is straight leg raising in the case of lordosis.

If the leg is raised to an angle of 90°, the already shortened psoas muscle is further contracted by exercising it, and accentuates the lordosed condition by an increased pull on the lumbar curve.

Exercise for the Abdominal Wall.—*Supine With Hands at the Side:* 1. Raise first one, then both feet (knee extended) from the floor just ten inches high. (This exercise is to stop before the psoas comes in to raise the leg farther. The abdominals act here to fix the pelvis.)

2. Flatten lower back against the floor, thus rotating the pelvis backward by contracting the abdominals.

3. Knees flexed, heels close to hips, lift hip and hold.

4. Same position as in 3 above, but now bring the flexed knees slowly over the chest and close to the face. This stretches the lower back muscles without bringing the psoas into use. Very useful in lordosis.

5. Same position as 3 and 4; now alternately bend and straighten the knees as in bicycle riding. Keep the hips off the floor.

6. Same position again, but now bring each knee alternately to the opposite shoulder. This strengthens the internal and external oblique muscles.

7. Supine lying: Have patient with each hand in turn forcibly push the operator's hand diagonally across the patient's body, first with right hand to left, then left hand to the right. This increases the strength of the internal oblique muscles. There can be felt a muscle tension in the upper quadrant on the same side.

Sitting Position: 1. Hands on hips, twist the body alternately to right and left, then change to hands on neck, arm shoulder high, then to arms over head.

2. Hands on hips, fix the pelvis and circumduct the trunk by bending the body forward, to the left, backwards, and to the right and forward again and up. Repeat in opposite direction.

3. Hands on the back of the neck, elbows back, reach high with the head, at the same time drawing abdominals upward. The elbows should be brought slowly and forcibly back with increasing effort. Not a pumping movement.

Standing Position: 1. Trunk flexion—bend the trunk alternately right and left without twisting, with hands first on the hips, then on the neck, and then with arms raised sidewise shoulder high. Avoid swaying the hips forward.

2. Trunk torsion—fix the hips firmly, using the body above the hips only, hands on hips, turn the trunk on its long axis alternately right and left.

3. Trunk circling—feet slightly apart, hands behind neck, fix

the hips and circumduct the trunk, first bending forward, to the right, backwards, to the left, and then again forward and up. Repeat all in the opposite direction.

MANAGEMENT BY EXERCISE OF THE UPPER BACK

Kyphosis.—This is an exaggerated posterior-anterior curvature of the dorsal portion of the spine. Round shoulders is the most common fault of posture, as nearly all occupations keep the head bent forward. Habitual round shoulders decrease respiration, hence lowering vitality, and favor various forms of deformity and disease. When round shoulders have become resistant and the subject can no longer assume the erect position, the condition is called kyphosis.

Corrective Exercises for Round Shoulders.—1. Patient lies supine with arms at sides, a small towel folded between the shoulder blades. Raise the arms forward and upward over the head while inhaling. Lower arms downward and forward to sides while exhaling.

2. Inhale while raising the head and chest from the floor with hands clasped behind the neck, elbows well back. Hold five counts. Exhale slowly while lowering head and chest.

3. With arms extended over the head, raise the arms, head and chest from the floor. Hold five counts, inhaling going up and exhaling coming down.

4. In sitting position, neck firm (hands are placed behind neck), stretch the head and chest and neck upward as far as possible, at the same time raising the elbows up to the maximum. Inhale going up, and exhale coming down.

5. In sitting position with hands clasped behind lower back, bring the shoulders together by pulling downward and inward with arms. Head is held back during the exercise. Caution: Do not allow hips to sway forward.

6. Stand facing a corner. With arms at shoulder level and the elbows bent at a 90° angle, place a hand on each wall. Inhale while pressing the chest into the corner. Keep abdominals tight. Exhale as the body is pushed out in returning to the original position.

MANAGEMENT BY EXERCISE OF THE LOWER BACK

Undetermined Chronic Back Pain.—The syndrome of chronic lower back pain is a common ailment characterized by chronicity and more or less disability. The type of lower backache to be mainly considered here is the one the pathology of which is not demonstrable by *X*-ray or clinical findings but which is disabling because of chronic pain. The pain is in all probability due to a spasm of the muscles and stress and strain of muscle, ligament, and joint in the area.

The immediate cause of pain may be explained as a result of overstimulation of proprioceptive stimuli arising within the muscle itself.

Rhythmical exercises are found to be of value in these cases where strengthening exercises would undoubtedly cause increased pain in muscles which are already in a state of hypertonicity and require relaxation. A good exercise for relaxation of the lower back is one described below. This exercise is found efficacious in conditions designated as sacro-iliac, lumbosacral, subluxation, or similar definitions denoting a disturbance of the lower back mechanism causing faulty coördination.

Relaxing Exercise for Lower Back Pain.—This exercise is performed by the patient taking a stride position, bending slightly forward and swinging rather than raising the arms. They should be held parallel with the hands several inches apart. Then by a twisting motion of the body, the arms are swung like a pendulum from one side to the other to a shoulder height. The arms are swung as a pendulum, not by means of the shoulder muscles but by lateral trunk bendings. As the arms are flung progressively higher, the body is turned from the hips in order to swing the arms above the head. This exercise is done slowly and rhythmically, preferably to music. The result of this exercise is the alternate contraction and relaxation of the right and left lower trunk muscles with the effect of slowly but gradually causing these muscles to respond to physiological inhibition. Also usable for this purpose are balancing movements.

Balance Exercise for Recoördination of Lower Back.—Begin balance steps by foot placing, progressing to swinging of the leg without touching the floor, and later adding bending of the supporting knee. These movements are calculated to correct the existing faulty coöordination and to relieve muscular spasm. They also tend to relieve the patient of an anxiety not to move his trunk either forward or laterally for fear that by doing so he might bring about the "old condition."

Lordosis.—Lordosis is an exaggerated anterior-posterior curvature of the lumbar portion of the spine. There is a shortening of the lower back muscles which may be due to a spasm of the muscles, or in later stages, to an actual contracture. This lower back condition varies and may be caused by several etiological factors.

1. Paralyzed or weakened abdominal muscles.
2. Paralyzed or weakened lower erector spinal muscles.
3. Faulty coöordination of trunk muscles.
4. Contracture of hip flexors or shortening of the iliofemoral ligament.
5. Faulty inclination of the pelvis.

The particular pathological condition must be ascertained before a plan for corrective exercises is formulated. If not carefully analyzed, the very treatment may exaggerate the condition instead of remedying it.

Patients with paralyzed abdominals present a lateral picture on standing, with the abdomen protruding markedly downward and forward, the lumbar curve exaggerated and a perpendicular line touching the gluteals and dorsal convexities. There is an inclination of the pelvis forward and downward, with shortening of the hip flexors. For this condition, many times incorrect "abdominal" exercises are prescribed. One of these, with the patient lying on the back and raising the straight leg upward to a 90° angle, is not an abdominal exercise, as it entails the use of the psoas hip flexor, which is already shortened and becomes increasingly so with exercising, thereby tending to exaggerate further the lumbar curve. (Note the position of the psoas muscle, its origin and insertion, arising from the sides of the bodies of all the lumbar vertebræ and inserting on the lesser trochanter of the femur.)

The exercise usually prescribed for the shortened back muscles is as follows: the patient lies supine, knees flexed, heels close to the buttocks, and hands resting on the sides near the hips. The exercise starts from this position. The patient slowly brings the knees up over the chest and as close to the face as possible, care being taken not to raise the head during the exercise. The patient slowly returns to the key position. The first part of the exercise should be performed with the patient exhaling to prevent the production of a possible hernia or a descent of the pelvic floor because of an increase in the intra-abdominal pressure.

Paralysis of the Lower Back Muscles.—If, with the lordotic condition, a marked weakening or even paralysis of the lower spinal muscles exists, the condition differs radically from the previously described one in which there is paralysis of the abdominals, and the treatment is accordingly different. When there is a paralysis of the lower spinal muscles, the patient presents a flat abdomen, with the upper part of his trunk leaning far backwards, so that a perpendicular line would touch the dorsal convexity. Compensating for a mechanical defect, the patient is trying to maintain balance in re-establishing his center of gravity by throwing his upper body backward to counteract the constant contracture of the opposing group, the abdominals and the psoas muscles, thus preventing flexion on the thighs. Here the problem is not to prescribe abdominal exercises but to make an effort to strengthen the lower spinal muscles. The following exercises may be given advantageously for this condition:

1. Lying prone, tighten the gluteal muscles. Hold ten counts.
2. Lying prone, straight leg extension, alternately and together.
3. Lying prone, grasp sides of bed with hands, cross right leg with left knee and repeat with opposite leg. This exercise rotates the lower part of the back.
4. Sitting with back straight, feet hooked under a chair rung, clasp the hands behind the neck, then lower the trunk backward. Make movement a slow and controlled one. Straighten up without emphasizing the forward movement.
5. Standing position; shrug one hip and extend the thigh on that side backward. Repeat on the other side. Do not turn or rotate the body with the hips.
6. Standing with the feet slightly apart, clasp hands behind the neck, bend trunk sideward; rotate trunk from side to side.

NOTE: The above six exercises are not to be given when there is a lordosis due to spasm or contracture of the muscles of the lower back.

It is quite evident that care is to be taken to distinguish between the three possible pathological conditions of the lower back: paralysis of the muscles of the lower back, spasm or contracture of the muscles of the lower back, and a shortening or spasm of these muscles due to a paralysis of the abdominal muscles.

MANAGEMENT BY EXERCISE OF BACK CURVATURES

Scoliosis, or Lateral Curvature of the Spinal Column.—The spinal column is an elastic, curved, segmented, weight bearing organ resting in an unstable position, and whereas its flexibility makes for great versatility of movement, it becomes automatically subject to various adverse strain or stress placed upon it.

Lateral curvature of the spine may involve either its entire length or one portion only of the vertebral column. The curve is usually in one direction only, but becomes "s" shaped since, to maintain body balance, a second compensatory curve in the opposite direction develops. Correction may be effected early, but if the vertebræ have become rotated, their shape permanently modified, the curvature finally becomes "fixed."

In only 5 per cent of all cases, including any condition which causes a tilting of the pelvis, can the cause be determined. Such conditions as chronic painful sacro-iliac joints, tuberculosis of the hip, talipes equinus, wryneck, empyema, poliomyelitis are the causative agents many times. Other causes are rickets, inanition causing muscular dystrophy in children under ten, habitual faulty postural habits as well as faulty occupational habits, manner of dress, chronic fatigue, and a timid apprehensive frame of mind causing a "psychoneurotic stance."

Scoliosis without apparent cause, the other 85 per cent, is four times as common in women as men, and in one-half of all cases it becomes evident between the ages of eleven and fifteen years.

Types of Scoliosis.—Lateral curvature, or scoliosis, is divided into two distinct classes: the structural and functional types.

The diagnosis of a structural curve is easily made by means of an *X*-ray; the findings show the wedge-shaped vertebræ in the apex of the curve, which in many instances is a right dorsal and is a secondary or compensatory curve to a primary left lumbar.

In a structural curve, muscles and ligaments have become shortened in the area of concavity and lengthened in the convexity. The patient cannot assume a corrected position with this type of scoliosis, and does not respond to correction by the means of exercise, but if a plaster cast or operative procedure is contemplated, preparatory exercise may be given to advantage in order to make the spine more flexible.

The functional curve (one in which the patient is able to assume a correct posture) responds very well to properly selected exercises.

Some of the features of an idiopathic structural scoliosis are these:

1. The convexity of the laterally deviated spine may be toward either the stronger or the weaker muscle side depending on which muscle groups are involved.

2. The convexity is toward the weak muscle side when the parallel bowstring muscles are weakened on the side of the convexity of the primary curve.

3. The concavity is toward the strong muscle side when the superficial transverse-traction-torsion muscles are weakened in the side of the convexity.

4. There is definite lateral deviation of the spine with relatively slight rotation of the bodies of the vertebræ when large superficial muscles are unbalanced.

5. There is rotation or torsion of the spine with relatively slight lateral displacement when deep intrinsic muscles of the spine are unbalanced.

There are evidently all combinations of unbalance involving eventually both the superficial and the deep intrinsic muscles of the spine where scoliosis is found.

Exercises for Scoliosis.—In cases of structural changes the exercises for scoliosis should be asymmetrical depending on the position of the lateral curvature. Passive manipulations may also be employed in this case. As correction is made, then symmetrical exercises may be given. If there is functional curvature, symmetrical exercises only are given.

If there is a deformity due to actual organic change, exercises are contraindicated, except those prescribed by physicians and those preceding operative procedures. Exercise may mobilize the spinal column, thereby increasing the curvature and instability of the spine, but may occasionally be prescribed for this purpose prior to plaster cast correction and surgical spinal fusion so that maximal correction may be obtained at the time of the operation.

Key or Basic Position for Exercises for Scoliosis:

1. Mobilization of the upper part of the back may best be obtained when it is bent forward.

2. Mobilization of the lower part of the back is best obtained when the upper part is extended back.

Correction of the Left Total Curvature of the Spine; Key Positions:

1. Lying prone with hands at side and the trunk and lower extremities deviated toward the side of the lumbar convexity, shrug the hip up on that side while raising the opposite arm high over the head and placing the other hand over the convexity.

2. Sitting on the edge of a chair so that the weight is on the hip and thigh of the side of the lumbar convexity, lower the opposite buttock by extending the thigh and leg backward. The upper part of the back is bent slightly forward. Now raise the opposite arm high over the head while the other hand covers and presses the side of convexity.

3. Kneeling on the side of the concavity, extend the opposite leg sideward. The upper back and arms the same as above in 2.

4. Crawling on the hands and knees, the knee on the side of the lumbar convexity is forward, and the opposite leg is stretched backward and inward. The arm on the side of the concavity is extended forward and inward, the other arm backward.

5. In standing position, lift the hip on the side of the lumbar convexity, raising the heel. Stretch the opposite arm high over the head, the other hand pressing on the convexity.

General posture exercises may be given in conjunction with the exercises given above.

GENERAL EXERCISES WHICH MAY BE GIVEN FOR REDUCTION OF HIPS AND ABDOMEN

1. Standing with one hand resting on a table or stall bar, the body held stiffly. Lift the leg opposite the supporting hand and with straight knee swing it backward and forward. Swing it out at the side. Swing in semi-circles. Repeat all with the opposite leg.

2. Standing with the feet a short distance apart, the arms at the sides. Without moving the shoulders or the feet, sway the hips from side to side. Make a circular movement with the hips over the feet as a central point.

3. Standing with the hands on the hips. Spring, and cross the feet, right and left, bringing each foot first in front of, then in behind the other.

4. Standing with the feet well apart, the hands on the hips. Sway the body slightly from side to side by using the muscles of the thighs and hips. Do not bend at the waist.

A possible error may be using the exercise as a "side bending" movement, and so using the muscles of the back and abdomen and not the thigh muscles.

NOTE: This exercise, like all exercises in which unusual muscle control is required, may require much patience and perseverance on the part of the patient and the instructor.

5. Standing. Raise the right leg with the knee bent, and grasp the knee with the left hand; then twist the body from side to side. Change and stand on the right foot, lifting the leg and twisting body.

6. Lying on the back, hands on hips with the legs extended and apart. Rotate the thighs in and out. Same position, swing the legs in, up, and out, making a semicircle, and back to rest position.

7. Lying on the back with the knees flexed. Separate the knees, giving resistance with the hands; bring them together again, resisting.

THE TEACHING OF POSTURE

Etiology of Faulty Posture.—A very common type of case coming to the physical medicine department is that of faulty postural habits.

Teaching posture in the past has rested largely on the supposition that poor posture was due to weak musculature, and elaborate systems of exercise were evolved, hoping to correct the condition. Now it is known that both theory and application were at fault.

It has been shown that there are many contributory causes of poor posture, such as faulty posture training given in schools and patterned after the old military concept of "shoulders back" and "toes out"; this along with poor seating facilities often paves the way for later poor postural habits.

In many cases, it is noted that the patient seems to be trying to get away from some discomfort, or at times, even pain, and tries to put to rest the particular part which is on strain. Together with these causes, functional etiology of faulty posture includes other factors.

It may be due to too rapid growth, improper clothing, style fads, and poor mental states. An example of this is the person having a mental attitude of depression or dejection achieving a slump posture, or the very arrogant person assuming a stiff inflexible posture, often the "hollow back" pathology. Also there are the very tall adolescents who try to decrease their height by slumping or stooping. This is more characteristic of girls than of boys.

Other causes of faulty posture are structural changes because of organic diseases, such as muscular or nervous weaknesses, injuries, arthritis, chronic backache, dysmenorrhea, rickets, and poor nutritional states and muscular dystrophies. These conditions having an organic foundation as a causative factor are partly pathological and require the guidance of medical physicians. Posture training is a secondary acquisition to the treatments. It may be well to add here that not only may disease cause poor posture, but faulty bodily alignment may well be the culprit in producing disease.

School surveys indicate that at least 75 per cent of our children carry themselves improperly with no improvement after thirty years. Soldiers of both world wars disclose a lamentable lack of physical fitness. These facts make evident the failure of our present physical educational system in a phase of endeavor distinctly within their scope.

The essential etiology of faulty posture, however, lies in an habitually assumed incorrect bodily attitude, allowing soft tissues, primarily muscular, to adapt themselves increasingly to the assumed position.

Correction is difficult, as shortened muscles resist stretching, and the lengthened muscles are too weak to function properly, thereby requiring a lengthy period of treatment in which weakened groups may be strengthened, and shortened groups may be stretched at the same time.

Another factor in the picture, frequently disregarded, is a discrepancy in the advancing development and relationship of the musculoskeletal and the neuromuscular apparatus, unfavorably affecting the kinesthetic sense. For example, a rapidly growing adolescent boy is awkward in his movements because he has a poor discriminative appreciation of spatial relationships and is therefore oblivious of grossly faulty positions.

Poor body mechanics present problems in mechanics and kinesiology which must be given due consideration in the plan for correction. Muscles which have become shortened because of adaptation to position are the calf, hamstrings, psoas, and lower back muscles, and the anterior shoulder girdle muscles. The weak and perhaps lengthened group comprise the anterior tibialis group, which normally support the long arch, the external rotators of the thigh, the gluteal group—especially the maximus and the abdominal muscles.

The above deficiencies produce such mechanical defects as pronated feet, anteriorly rotated pelvis, lordosis, round shoulders, depressed anterior thorax and sagging of the abdominal contents. We believe that the chief offender is the rotated pelvis. Thus stretching, strengthening muscles and training in balance and poise must extend to all parts of the body in any plan for correcting faulty body mechanics.

Mechanics of the Erect Posture.—Good posture has once been defined as the mechanical correlation of the various systems of the body with their special reference to the skeletal, muscular, and visceral systems and their neurological associations.

This position obtains when the feet, the lower extremities, the pelvis, the trunk and the head are aligned so as to produce a minimum of effort, tension, and strain in the endeavor to maintain erect bodily carriage.

This upright position is held by a sense of balance, keeping the center of gravity over the center of support. Balance and the upright position depend on three kinds of sensory stimuli which act on motor neurons of all muscles to regulate tension: (1) stimuli from the semicircular canals; (2) stimuli from the eyes; and (3) stimuli from proprioceptive centers in muscles, tendons and ligaments aid in maintaining an erect position. It may be added that stimuli from sensory cells of the skin, especially from the soles of the feet, also contribute in this phenomenon.

The prime necessities for acquiring and maintaining correct carriage are these: (1) Maintenance of health and vitality by proper living habits. (2) Conservation of energy, ability to relax and rest (including recreation). (3) Prevention of postural habits, correction of faulty habits, training in habits of coördination, and the maintenance of corrected erect posture.

Theories of Mechanics of Erect Posture.—There are several theories concerning the correct attitude for erect posture which involve the straight line test and the establishment of the center of gravity. It is assumed by some that the tilt of the pelvis should be on an angle of 55° to 60°, but this being impossible to measure, the normal tilt is considered to be one in which a line extending between the anterior-superior spines of the iliac bones is directly over the symphysis pubis. Any straight line test should find that the ear shoulder, hip, knee, and a point just anterior to the ankle should be in a vertical plane.

Various theories for pelvic tilt are as follows:

1. Lovett-Reynolds: The center of gravity is in front of the hip.

2. McKenzie: In normal standing position, the long axis of the head and neck and trunk and legs form a straight line. Center of gravity is in front of ankle joint. Pelvis tilt should be at a 30° angle.

3. Bowen-McKenzie: All body segments from head to ankle form an approximately straight line, which is inclined forward from the ankles on the balls of the foot. Pelvis tilt should be at a 60° angle.

4. Bancroft agrees with Bowen.

5. Trislow and Dickinson: The line of gravity passes through important pivotal points. The rear perpendicular touches two points, the shoulder and the buttocks.

6. Goldthwait: To hold the body so that it is made as tall as possible, without rising on toes. Pelvic tilt should be at a 30° angle.

7. The authors believe that to attain a correct postural habit, one must stand erect and move the trunk forward so that most of the weight is on the balls of the feet, and only a very slight swaying forward is necessary to enable the patient to raise his heels off the floor. The pelvis should be rotated backward on a line with the symphysis pubis.

Management of Posture by Exercise.—The use of exercise to reconstruct postural defects, after an analysis of the patient's needs are ascertained, usually begins with attention to the feet and then to other parts of the body in a definite plan for postural re-education.

The Feet.—The feet are placed parallel and about four or five inches apart, with the weight mainly on the forepart of the feet.

The Hips.—Attention is next directed to the fact that the hips must be brought backward. During the analysis it may be found the hips are too far forward. An attempt is made to explain that what is desired is a tilting of the pelvis upward and backward.

Various methods are used to produce this result; for examples a mental picture of trying to squeeze sidewards between two board,

7

with less distance between them than the anterior-posterior diameter of the individual is found helpful. This should cause the symphysis to rise and the gluteals to lower with the desired result. Moving back the pelvis places the hips in their proper position and corrects the lordosis.

The Trunk.—What is desired is a rotation of the trunk on an axis midway between shoulder and hip which will in reality bring the hips backward and the upper half of the trunk forward. We cannot use the phrase "throw out your chest" because this invariably leads to an exaggerated chest position plus a lordosis. The command is to "raise your chest," and avoid the terms "chest out" or "shoulder back." We get the patient to raise the back part of his head (the occiput) by asking him to imagine that he is trying to touch the ceiling with this part of his head.

Balance.—The proper distribution of the body weight on the feet offers opportunity to explain the cause of poor mechanics. An undue proportion of body weight on the heels causes a compensatory forward movement of the hips for the purpose of sustaining balance. This leads to a second compensatory movement, a rounding of the shoulders with corresponding forward movement of the head, the total producing a typical fatigue posture, spoken of diagrammatically as the zig-zag position. The prime consideration is the proper distribution of the weight on the feet, achieved by transferring a considerable portion of the weight to the ball of the foot. This adjustment of weight with hips, chest, and head corrected as outlined, enables the patient to raise his heels off the floor, causing the body to move straight upward without a forward swaying motion the "test position." Whether or not the patient can raise his heels off the floor without a forward motion of the body may be ascertained by placing one's finger in front of his shoulder, and if he sways forward past the finger, this is an indication that he had first to transfer his weight from his heels before he could raise them from the floor. This raising of the heels forms the basis of our habit-forming process, as well as being the test for distribution of the weight on the feet.

Teaching Method.—On the theory that repetition produces a habit, the patient is repeatedly asked to assume the corrected posture, and to test his position by raising the heels. It is much to be preferred that all teaching be done in front of a long mirror so that he can see the process being carried out. If the patient is a child, it is preferable that the mother should attend the posture demonstration and learn the proper method of instruction for the child.

Exercises.—It must not be assumed that correction can be obtained without some exercises. These are selected mainly for the purpose of stretching some, shortening other, muscles, and, through the awakening of the kinesthetic sense, conveying to the patient a clearer mental picture of the position to be attained. The importance of selection lies in recognizing these factors:

1. The upper anterior chest muscles and ligaments must be stretched.

2. The lower back muscles, which have become shortened because of the lordotic position, must be stretched.

3. The hip flexors must not be strengthened. A typical error is made by asking the patient to raise the extended legs 90° while lying on the floor. This exercises the abdominal muscles but little, merely to the extent of fixing the pelvis so that the extended legs can be brought to a 90° angle by action of the hip flexors. With a tilting of the pelvis forward there is not only a protuberant abdomen, but also a lordosis, and a physiological shortening of the hip flexors, tending thereby to hold the pelvis in the acquired forward tilting position. It follows that a further strengthening of the hip flexors defeats the purpose. For this reason care must be taken not to choose an exercise which forcibly brings into action the hip flexors.

When other factors as general muscular weakness, improper clothing, and ill-chosen chairs and beds are contributory causes of faulty posture, general all around exercises are indicated.

1. Exercise to stretch shortened muscles of the chest.
   (*a*) Patient lying on his back with a pillow or folded towel between his shoulder blades, arms extended sideward shoulder high. Patient should hold this position for five to ten minutes, two or three times daily.
   (*b*) Patient stands, takes the corrected posture position, and places both hands on his neck. Bring the elbows as far backward as possible and at the same time sway the entire body well forward. Raise the heels off floor and pull hard on the elbows.

NOTE: The importance of this exercise lies in the fact that it is a continuous pulling of the elbows back for as long a time as possible. A common error is a tendency to sway the hips forward the harder the elbows are pulled backward. Therefore, care must be exercised in counteracting the tendency of the forward swing of the hips.

The exaggerated position assumed while taking this exercise stimulates the kinetic sense by arousing sensory impulses in skin, muscles, tendons and articular surfaces, thereby producing for the individual a clearer mental picture of the posture desired.

2. Exercise for mild abdominal contraction.
   (*a*) Patient lying on his back, raises the extended legs ten inches only from the floor.
   NOTE: This exercise fixes the pelvis and makes impossible hip flexion by restricting leg raising to 10° only.
3. Exercise to strengthen and shorten abdominal muscles.
   (*a*) Patient lying on his back, comes to a half-sitting position.
   (*b*) Patient lying on his back, knees bent, and heels close to the body, brings both knees as close to the head as possible. Return to starting position.
   NOTE: This exercise forcibly shortens the abdominal group and reverses the lordotic curve.
4. Exercise to strengthen the abdominal muscles.
   (*a*) Lying supine with knees flexed, feet flat on the floor, inhale and exhale while flattening the back on floor.
   (*b*) Have patient stand a little distance from a wall with the back of the shoulders and hips touching the wall, then flatten the lower back against the wall.

Final Instructions.—The patient is instructed to take the exercises described above two or three times daily, if possible before a mirror, or before some one who knows the proper posture instructions. He is asked to assume the corrected position once every hour, and check himself by heel raising (posture test).[1] This is extremely important as it underlies the whole scheme of posture training. It aids materially in creating a new postural sense by causing the individual to become "posture minded or posture conscious."

The patient is asked to return after several days and at subsequent intervals as conditions may necessitate for a check-up. Two or more instruction periods, depending upon the intelligence and coöperation of the individual, may be required for the patient to master the instructions.

[1] Page 98.

CHAPTER VIII

APPLICATION OF THERAPEUTIC EXERCISE IN MEDICINE

CARDIAC DISEASE

THE effect of exercise on the heart is unfortunately not well understood by the general practitioner. The usual procedure, to restrain the patient from all activities, in some instances is damaging to the individual as a whole and should be avoided whenever possible.

In certain cardiac diseases definite improvement results from the prescription of proper exercise. In both normal and cardiac patients dyspnea is the greatest safeguard against possible heart strain or cardiac failure; therefore, a program should be planned based on the capacity of the heart to respond to effort as manifested by the absence of dyspnea.

1. *Master's Test:* The "Master's Test," or tolerance test for circulatory efficiency, should precede a system of general exercise for cardiac disease. The patient climbs steps in which he is required to take two steps up and two down consecutively in climbing over the device. Thus, he is forced to take turns first to the right and then to the left as he goes back and forth over the steps for ninety seconds. His blood pressure and pulse are taken before and after and then checked with a table predetermined for age, weight, and sex. A return of the rate to within five beats of the pulse before the exercise and to not more than five millimeters mercury in blood pressure is considered normal if these occur within two minutes.

2. *August Schott Exercises:* Perhaps the first scientifically planned exercises were originated by August Schott and his brother. These are based upon the heart's capacity to respond to exercise, and the absence of dyspnea.

The exercises are characterized by three factors: (*a*) They are mildly resistive. (*b*) They must be performed very slowly (so slowly as to tax the operator's patience). (*c*) They must fall short of fatigue, the early symptoms of which must be carefully noted.

Each movement must take no less than one-half minute, followed by one-half minute rest before the next movement is begun. The exercises are mainly slightly resistive ones, unless the case is severe, in which case the movements are passive until the patient can perform without fatigue. The patient may take his exercises in bed at first, in which case joint motions are performed for him; then he may progress to a sitting position for exercises and finally may be able to take them standing. Various types may be given, such as abdominal, foot or breathing exercises.

3. *The Oertel Terrain Cure:* If the patient is an ambulatory one, he may have prescribed for him the terrain cure, a plan in which the patient may walk for a definitely prescribed distance and back to the starting point, the distance being gradually increased with the increased tolerance of the patient for exercise.

PERIPHERAL VASCULAR DISEASE

Exercise has been found to be beneficial in many cases of peripheral vascular disease. The following exercises are used frequently in occlusive vascular disease.

1. The patient lies on his back. The leg is elevated to nearly 90° during which time it is either supported by a sling or held by the patient or by an attendant for from thirty seconds to three minutes according to the time required to produce blanching. It is then lowered over the side of the bed until the skin of the foot and legs become reddened, signifying a hyperemia. The leg is permitted to remain in this hanging position for a minute longer, provided the patient can tolerate it, and is then returned to the resting horizontal position on the bed for a period equal to the time consumed in elevating and lowering the leg. During this time heat may be applied. The duration of the cycle (comprising elevation, lowering and resting the leg) varies with each patient and should be repeated four to six times during the day. The leg is allowed complete rest for at least an hour between exercise cycles.

2. Various devices have been developed for improvement of the circulation in the extremities; one of the most commonly used is the suction-pressure boot. The pressure in the boot (usually made of glass) is alternated so that there are a prescribed number of seconds of negative pressure and a prescribed number of seconds of positive pressure. It is frequently set at twenty-five seconds of negative pressure at 80 to 120 mm. mercury, and five seconds of positive pressure at 20 to 80 mm. mercury. Many variations of the duration of these pressures may be employed.

HEMIPLEGIA

One week after the onset of the paralysis, the patient may be taken through joint motions, but passive exercises in which the patient is asked to coöperate are employed, so that muscle re-education may be started early. As soon as function begins to return, the patient is encouraged to attempt some voluntary movements. It should be kept in mind that all exercises given to strengthen the weaker group should tend to stretch the stronger spastic group. The extremities are to be in a neutral or physiological rest position when the patient is not exercising. Coördination of parts is sought early by rhythmic movements. The exercises are done in a routine manner, re-educating each segment in turn. The patient is instructed to endeavor to maintain each movement at its completion for a brief period before it is allowed to relax, while the adjacent segment is being exercised. Strong effort at extension of all joints is to be stressed.

Exercises are first given in the early treatments with the patient in a reclining position, then in a sitting position after some motion has been obtained. Later he probably will have attained a walking position and have need of balance and foot placing exercises. Preceding walking, proper attention should have been given to flexion and extension of the hips and knees and the muscles producing these actions should have reached the "fair" status.

AFFECTIONS OF THE SEVENTH NERVE

The path of the seventh nerve (a mixed nerve, mainly motor) is from the fourth ventricle through the inner ear, emerging in front of the external auditory canal, and passing through the substance of the parotid gland.

The branches of the seventh nerve supply all the muscles of the face except the muscles of mastication, and pathology of this nerve may cause a paralysis of the facial muscles.

Conditions which may affect the seventh nerve:

Traumatic Type:

1. Fracture of skull, tumors, hemorrhage.
2. Mastoid operations in which the seventh nerve is severed or injured.
3. Wounds or severe blows to the face.

If the lesion is due to cerebral hemorrhage, pressure of a new growth or other pathological condition of the brain, the cause of the facial paralysis lies within the cerebrum (above the pons) and the frontalis, corrugator and orbicularis oculi muscles are not affected. The patient can raise his eyebrows, wrinkle his forehead and close his eye.

However, this condition is of more serious import because it is accompanied by a paralysis of the abducens; a hemiplegia of the opposite side of the body will be manifested as well.

Rheumatic Type: Bell's palsy.

The pathology consists of a peripheral neuritis of the nerve trunk following exposure to cold or to a chilling draft. It is quite possible that a pre-existing focal infection was a predisposing factor.

Seventy-five per cent of all facial nerve lesions fall into the group of Bell's palsy. The paralysis is of the flaccid type, and occurs on the affected side, which appears mask-like. Other symptoms besides paralysis are the following:

1. Food collection between the cheeks and the gums.
2. A flow of tears from the affected eye.
3. Possible loss of deep facial sensation.
4. Possible loss of taste in the anterior two-thirds of tongue.
5. Reduced salivation on the affected side.
6. Possible associated pain because of involvement of other nerves (trigeminal, auditory, etc.).

After about ten days there should be given a test for reaction of degeneration. Treatment should be initiated as soon as possible, consisting of daily short exposures to infra-red radiation and muscle re-education. The physician may prescribe light dosages of electrical stimulation.

SEVENTH NERVE FACIAL MUSCLE CHART

(Branches of the seventh nerve supply all facial muscles except muscles of mastication.)

7th Nerve Branch	*Muscle Supplied*	*Muscle Function*	*Exercise (assistive)*
	(The buccal nerve supplies the muscles of the nose and upper lips.)		
Buccal nerve	1. Compressor naris	1. Raises wing of nose.	1. Have patient try to dilate nostrils
	2. Risorius	2. Draws lips laterally to express pain	2. Have patient try to stretch lips sideward
	3. Buccinator	3. Flattens cheeks against teeth, as in whistling	3. Have patient try to whistle
	4. Incisivus	4. Draws corners of lips medially	4. Have patient try to pull corners of mouth together.
	5. Orbicularis oris	5. Purses lips	5. Have patient try to pucker lips
	6. Triangularis	6. Draws lips laterally as in grief	6. Have patient try to draw lips laterally and slightly upward
Mandibular nerve	1. Quadratus labii inferior	1. Draws lower lips downward	1. Have patient try to curl lips downward
	2. Mentalis	2. Draws up the skin of chin	2. Have patient try to wrinkle chin
Temporal nerve	1. Orbicularis oculi	1. Closes eyelids	1. Have patient try to close eyelids
	2. Corrugator	2. Draws brows together	2. Have patient try to frown
	3. Procerus	3. Draws skin of forehead across root of nose (between the eyes)	3. Have patient try to draw brows together and downward
	4. Frontalis	4. Elevates eyebrows	4. Have patient simulate surprise
Zygomaticus nerve	1. Quadratus labii superior	1. Raises lateral half of upper lips and wing of nose	1. Have patient try to smile
	2. Caninus	2. Raises corners of upper lips and at the same time draws them medially	2. Have patient try to sneer or express bitterness
	3. Zygomaticus	3. Draws mouth forcibly sideward and upward	3. Have patient try to laugh

ARTHRITIS

In the administration of exercise for persons suffering with joint disturbances, it is, of course, essential that discrimination and judgment are used with respect to types of exercise, such as weight bearing, fatigue, dosage, time of day, and other factors. No motion should be attempted during the acute stage. When this has passed, however, a carefully planned régime of heat, massage, and movement may be instituted properly, the object being not only to give attention to the negative phase of preventing atrophy of the muscle, but also to direct positive attention to improving the existing condition. Mobilization of the joint is necessary to prevent ankylosis and adhesions. Movement stimulates circulation and improves nutrition of the tissue.

The selection of the type of exercise is made from passive, assistive, and active. Sling suspension exercises, muscle setting, and non-weight-bearing active exercises may be given. Care must be taken from the beginning not to add to heart strain in these patients. Transition is gradually made from simple formal movements to purposeful active exercises such as walking, swimming, and occupational therapy measures. If swimming is attempted, the water should preferably be 98° Fahrenheit.

TABES DORSALIS

The following exercises are especially arranged for use in tabes dorsalis and other diseases which involve the reflex mechanism controlling proprioceptive impulses from muscles, tendons, and joints; conditions which confuse finely coördinated movements because the sense of position, the appreciation of the spatial relationship of one part of the body to another has been altered. The movements, therefore, are characterized by being purposeful, discerning, and volitional. Repetition of exact movements is the keynote of the exercises. They are designed not to strengthen muscles but to educate them to act as directed. Control and coördination are to be sought after in performance of the exercises assigned. Some of the following exercises may be given for this disease.

Supine With Arms Beside Body.

(*a*) Alternate flexion and extension of knee and hip.

(*b*) Abduction and adduction with knee bent.

(*c*) Abduction and adduction with knee straight.

(*d*) With the toe of one foot, touch the other leg at knee, at ankle, and at toe. Repeat with the other foot.

(*e*) Flex and extend both legs at the same time, knees and ankles close together; extend the feet through an opening (ring, etc.) without allowing the feet to touch the sides of the ring. Repeat all the above with the eyes closed.

Sitting Position.

(*a*) Patient places his foot in the hand of the operator who changes the position of the hand each time.

(*b*) With heels close together, patient rises from a chair to a standing position, slowly and deliberately. This aids in acquiring motor control and attaining body balance.

(*c*) Foot-placing exercises devised by marking footprints on the floor require the patient to try to place his feet deliberately in the chalked prints.

Standing Position.

(*a*) The patient raises one knee, places the foot firmly on the floor in traced footprints. Repeat forward, sideward, and backward.

(*b*) The patient walks on two parallel lines, chalked on the floor six inches apart; then follows markings along a zigzag line.

(*c*) If the upper extremities are affected, writing and drawing are helpful. When the patient has practiced writing at a table, he is then taught to increase the size of his writing on a blackboard, changing in this manner from a horizontal to a vertical one, and from finger movements to arm movements.

(*d*) Finger pointing at spots of interest on a map aids in teaching coördination of the upper extremity.

These exercises follow the theory that when sensation has departed from the extremities, the patient only through the use of other senses controls their movements. When a tabetic patient becomes blind (some patients develop optic atrophy), he loses sensation in his legs as well as the sighted patient; but having lost the use of the eyes, all other sensory tracts are so thoroughly developed that they compensate in an effective substitute for vision; then as the controlling arcs are still within the body, the ataxia is less marked than if a portion of the arc were outside the body in respect to sensations. Certainly if it is possible for a blind tabetic to master his ataxia by the instinctive training of other senses, it is equally possible to teach a sighted patient to do likewise. It is essential to begin re-education of the finer movements before the grosser ones are fully mastered.

RESPIRATORY CASES

In asthmatic conditions the patient has most difficulty in expiration, especially during an attack. The chronic sufferers have respiration almost entirely of the upper thoracic cage, the lower part of the thorax remaining fully expanded with diaphragmatic excursions very slight. Accordingly, it is desirable to inhibit upper and to encourage lower thoracic breathing. To prevent undue distension of the lungs, the use of the lower portion of the thorax and diaphragm is stressed. By the proper exercise as the patient learns that he can control an attack of asthma, his fear of having an attack is greatly lessened. Before the following exercises are given, several preliminary measures should be considered: (1) The patient is first instructed to clear the nasal passages. (2) Each exercise should be preceded by a short, gentle inspiration through the nose, followed by forced expiration through the mouth. (3) During inspiration the upper thorax is immobilized. (4) During expiration, the abdominals should be contracted ("pulled in"). This phase is continued as long as possible.

(*a*) *Abdominal Breathing:* Supine with knees drawn up, body relaxed, the hand on the upper abdomen, the patient exhales slowly, sinking his chest, and then the upper abdomen. Now holding the chest down, he relaxes the upper abdomen, taking in gentle inspiration and repeating the expiration. Repeat cycle eight to ten times.

(*b*) *Side Expansion Breathing:* Sitting relaxed (the lower thorax is confined with a belt), the patient exhales slowly, first with the upper and then with the lower thorax; then tightening the lower ribs with the belt, he inhales quietly, compressing the ribs against the belt. The arms and shoulders are relaxed. Repeat with further tightening of the belt, a little at a time, each time within the patient's tolerance.

NOTE: For children, follow the same procedure, substituting the child's own hands for compression of the ribs instead of the belt.

(*c*) *Elbows Describing a Circle* (this exercise is to be performed between breathing exercises): Standing, the patient leans forward with the hips and back straight, and fingers on the shoulders, elbows back and at shoulder level. The elbows are circled forward, upward, backward, and downward while the patient rises on toes and straightens back. Lowering the heels, the patient repeats cycle four to six times.

(*d*) *Forward Bending:* Sitting with the feet together and arms relaxed at the sides, exhaling slowly, dropping the head forward, the patient brings his knees up to his chest, clasping them with his arms, and bends back until the head is over the knees. The abdominals are contracted firmly. He inspires while uncurling the trunk and expands the abdomen; he exhales quickly, sitting with the chest and abdomen compressed. Next he inhales slightly, expanding the upper part of the abdomen only. Repeat all four to six times.

Other breathing exercises may be given for various conditions.

In inactive tuberculosis, as it is desirable that thoracic breathing should be minimized as much as possible, abdominal breathing is thus encouraged.

In other conditions, such as posture with a protruding abdomen, a forward upward chest elevation with shoulders relaxed and a lateral spread of the lower rib cage are the essential points to be stressed in breathing. A good exercise which does all this is as follows:

Lying supine with hands on top of the head or at the back of the neck and knees bent:

1. Breathe deeply, raising the chest, keeping lower back down to the floor.
2. Exhale by drawing the lower abdomen in, keeping the chest lifted.
3. Inhale again, holding the chest position.
4. Exhale again, using the lower abdomen alone.

The amount of breath passing in this exercise is not important. The two important points are the constantly lifted chest, higher with each inhalation, and, second, the exhalation by inward-upward contraction of the lower abdomen.

Breathing exercises may be given for maintaining fitness to the normal healthy individual who cannot endure vigorous exercises, or to those who are hindered from it by conditions which make active exercise impossible. These individuals are given voluntary deep breathing exercises. The extent to which it is possible to gain control of the individual muscles of breathing so as to inhale and exhale in a variety of ways is surprising. They find it possible also to learn to breathe in ways that will accord with the movement being made, and to economize nervous and muscular force.

Mobility of the chest is a factor quite as much as size in the measurement of efficiency of the lungs. With a mobile chest the muscles can more easily move the amount of air needed in quiet breathing. Accordingly, the patient extends his ability to endure exercise.

CHAPTER IX

POLIOMYELITIS

ACUTE ANTERIOR (EPIDEMIC INFANTILE PARALYSIS) AND CHRONIC ANTERIOR POLIOMYELITIS

Evaluation of the Disease.—In the treatment of poliomyelitis it is important that its several forms and their variations are recognized. Acute anterior or epidemic infantile paralysis shows symptoms which, except for paralysis, are very similar to other infections of the nervous system, especially to meningitis. The effect of the acute anterior type upon the patient may fall into any one of these categories: (1) total incapacitation during the period of systemic infection with speedy recovery and no appreciable residual effects; (2) negligible or even undetectable symptoms from which the patient recovers without residual muscular weaknesses; and (3) total incapacitation with fatal result, as in cases involving the muscles of respiration and deglutition. The first and second types are classed as "abortive" and are curable by one or another form of treatment.

In *chronic anterior poliomyelitis* the period of paralysis continues beyond convalescence, *i. e.*, from one and one-half to two years after the onset. This condition is sometimes referred to as "progressive spinal muscular atrophy." The motor cells of the cord disappear; their fibers in the peripheral motor nerves become functionally inactive and eventually are absorbed. The resultant slow atrophy of muscles is indicated in the early stage by a fine twitching of their fibers or "fibrillary twitching."

This paralysis may be extensive or possibly limited to a few muscles of one or more extremities, often to only parts of muscles; it may involve the face, the diaphragm, or the intercostal muscles. In a child who has sustained total paralysis of all the muscles of an extremity, the member fails to develop normally and remains shorter and more shrunken than its mate. It is weak, limp and flaccid (flail-like). If only part of the muscles of the limb are affected, a marked deformity may be present on account of the unopposed pull of a normal muscle against its paralyzed opponent. This illustrates one type of "club foot" as well as many cases of scoliosis otherwise unexplained.

This type of paralysis shows none of the consistent patterns or "systems" common to other types of paralysis (as in hemiplegia) but displays a "patchy" or scattered pattern.

Anatomical Consideration of Poliomyelitis.—In the anterior horn of the cord lie the nerve cells, the fibers of which form the peripheral motor nerves. If a motor fiber is injured, a new one will grow from the cell to take its place, but if the motor cell dies, its function is never in any way restored, and its fiber, together with the muscle fiber which it controls, likewise will die. This injury is permanent.

Accompanying the invasion of the nervous system by the virus, inflammation in the spinal cord is most active. Although the chief residual effect is upon the anterior horn cell, the inflammation is not limited to that area, as all parts of the cord may be involved, including the meninges.

Frequently it is noted that after the period of inflammation has passed, there is a relatively rapid period of recovery when muscle re-education is aptly administered. However, if no treatment or if improper treatment is administered, the muscles may become atrophied from disuse as the habit patterns once followed by the neuromuscular mechanism are estranged from the higher center because of the inability of the muscles to perform their accustomed motions during the period of inflammatory process extending throughout the motor paths. Thus, atrophy may occasionally occur even in the presence of relatively little damage to the cell itself. This damage is then due to wasting of the muscles from disuse and is directly attributable to a physiological break in the old-established motion patterns, and not to a direct organic lesion of the cell itself.

The paralysis following damage to the anterior horn cell and its fibers is of the flaccid type. However, the lesion may occur in the upper neuron with an involvement of the pyramidal tracts in the inflammatory processes, giving rise to spasm in some muscle or group of muscles.

Evaluation of Treatment of Poliomyelitis.—With the divergence of medical aspects of poliomyelitis and the resultant uncertainty of diagnosis in the early stages, the evaluation of treatment is very difficult. The possibility of instituting early treatment is unfortunately limited by the time element involved in securing accurate diagnosis.

Although it is not feasible to begin a program of re-education during the acute systemic manifestation of the disease, an early diagnosis is desirable for applying hot moist packs, splinting, and the use of a respirator, if the need arises.

Accuracy of diagnosis, although not easily attainable, is very desirable and recognition of this fact should serve to avoid confusion occurring not only from the multiplicity of possible individual symptoms, but also from the "degree of severity" of the infection which may take form in a single epidemic from negligible or even undetectable symptoms in one patient to a rapidly fatal issue in another.

Evaluation of treatment of the various manifestations of poliomyelitis, therefore, should be made in consideration of the severity of the "residual muscular weaknesses" and treatment of "abortive cases" should not be a "norm" for establishing a reputation for any particular form of treatment in comparison with treatment in cases in which the residual paralysis continues after the acute stages of the disease. Therefore, for fair comparison of any two forms of treatment an equal sampling of cases is necessary.

Treatment must also take into account the various aspects of the disease accompanying the residual paralysis. Resocialization and rehabilitation of the individual as a whole organism should join the re-education measures as a triad of therapeutics for physical, psychic, and social sequels which accompany the convalescence of this disease.

TREATMENT DURING THE ACUTE STAGES

Testing by Topographical Observation as a Preliminary Measure for the Administration of Hot Packs.—1. **Evaluation of Muscle Spasm.**—Accurate evaluation of muscles or muscle groups in spasm is made possible by topographical scrutinization during the acute stage of poliomyelitis *before* it is expedient to ascertain muscle function by the volitional test and as a preliminary measure for the administration of hot foments.

After the period of pain and inflammatory processes in the muscle has passed, a volitional muscle function test may be performed, preferably in water, to establish the status of the muscle as a guide for a plan of muscle re-education.

The following points for observation are presented:

"The occurrence of inflammatory processes may be noted by observation of abnormal skin creases, prominence of muscle bellies or tendons, and characteristic positions assumed by the particular part. Occasionally the physician is able to locate the spasm by observation and some palpation without necessarily encouraging any painful motions. The spasm is carefully stretched passively to diminish it for diagnostic purposes. It is imperative not to aggravate the condition by overenthusiastic manipulation during this stage.

"Occurrence of spasm; spasm is usually found most frequently in the following order:

1. Hamstring muscles
2. Back and neck muscles
3. Calf muscles
4. Pectorals
5. Muscles of respiration
6. Quadriceps muscle
7. Biceps of the arm

"*Neck Region:* Inspection may show a prominence of the extensor group (posteriorly) showing a deep cleft between them. Observe if the head is pulled back in hyperextension. Note the anterior aspect of the neck for sternocleidomastoideus. Spasm in one will turn the face toward the opposite side. Spasm in both will pull the face downward in flexion.

"*Shoulder Girdle:* A spasm in the pectoralis major is often shown by the presence of several creases at the anterior axillary line, and a forward angulation of the head of the humerus resulting in a cupped shoulder. Note whether shoulders are elevated on either side as there may be spasm of either one of the levator scapulæ or upper trapezius.

"*The Arm:* Spasm in the biceps is shown by inability to extend the elbow in 180°. Biceps tendon stands out. The belly of the muscle is more prominent than normal.

"*The Forearm:* Spasm in the flexor group is shown by flexed position of the fingers and hand. Spasm in the long flexors and extensors of the fingers and abductors of the thumb may be indicated by prominence of the respective tendons. Spasm in the supinators or pronators is shown by limitation of motion and pain in carrying out the opposite action.

"*The Hand:* Spasm in the opponens pollicis is shown by tenderness in the belly of the muscle and inability to abduct the thumb.

"Spasm in the interossei and lumbricales is shown by stiffness of the fingers.

"*The Back* (trunk muscles): Spasm in the back muscles is evidenced by pain, stiffness, and inability to flex the back actively or passively, and may be so severe as to cause a lordosis or an opisthotonos, or so painful as to make a supine position unendurable for more than a few minutes. This spasm may be localized to various areas or to either side, resulting in a scoliosis and other deformities. The erector spinæ group is not usually prominent but is flattened and narrowed by spasm. The spine is curved with the concavity toward the spasm. If there is extensive spasm in the back, the abdominals are 'alienated.'

"Spasm in the intercostals causes interference with respiration and is evidenced by a depressed or elevated thoracic cage. The pectoralis major is in spasm in sympathy with the intercostals.

"Spasm in the diaphragm may be shown by a depression in the lower rib, a groove around the chest, and an elevated chest, and the difficulty is with expiration and not with inspiration.

"Spasm in the lateral abdominals causes apparent shortening of one leg by elevation of the pelvis on that side and the anterior superior iliac spine may be prominent on that side.

"Spasm in the psoas may cause flexion at the hips and pain on hyperextension of the thighs.

"Spasm in the rectus abdominis is shown by an exaggerated groove over the linea alba.

"*The Hip and Thigh:* Spasm in the gluteus maximus may cause external rotation of the thigh and prominence of the involved muscle or, in the extreme case, the natal cleft may be widened.

"Spasm in the hamstrings may be more marked in the inner or outer sides. The knees may be held in a slightly flexed position putting the quadriceps on the stretch.

"Spasm in the tensor fascia lata is shown by a tight band on the lateral surface of the thigh toward the knee.

"Spasm of the quadriceps is shown by inability to flex the knee without pain and prominence of the muscles involved, especially the rectus femoris.

"Spasm of the sartorius is shown by a prominence in the region of the anterior superior spine of the ilium. The leg may be externally rotated, accompanied by a lordosis by pulling the pelvis forward.

"Spasm in the adductors is shown by tenseness in the medial portion of the thigh and inability to abduct the leg without pain to those muscles.

"*The Leg:* Spasm is commonly found in the calf muscles (gastrocnemius and soleus muscles). If in the lateral head, the heel is everted. If spasm occurs in the medial head, the heel is inverted. The whole foot is plantar flexed as shown by a 'foot drop.' Spasm in the posterior tibial is shown by a tendinous ridge just posterior to the medial malleolus.

"In the anterior aspect of the leg, spasm is shown by prominence of the muscle tendons of the involved muscles and a calcaneus position of the foot if there is no accompanying spasm in the calf.

"*The Foot:* Spasm in the intrinsic muscles of the foot is shown by deformities of the toes (pes cavus), or pain in stretching."[1]

[1] Cole, W. H., Pohl, J. F. and Knapp, M. E.: "The Kenny Method of Treatment for Infantile Paralysis," New York, The National Foundation for Infantile Paralysis, Inc., Pub. 40, 1942.

Treatment of Muscle Spasm by Hot Foments.—As soon as spasm is diagnosed treatment is started by the use of hot foments, which are placed accurately over the areas in which spasm is located. They are usually renewed every two hours, but may be applied more often if the spasm is severe. The packs are continued uninterruptedly, being changed as indicated throughout twelve hours of the day. Occasionally it is found necessary to continue them during the night if the patient is in severe pain.

The foments are boiled and wrung from the boiling water so that as much water as possible is removed. There should be no burns if the water is well expelled from the packs. A machine is now ordinarily used, having a centrifugally operated drum which expels excess water from the packs and leaves them moist and hot. The packs must be applied hot but dry enough to prevent burning. The packs may be boiled for twenty minutes if sterilization is needed, otherwise they are just heated thoroughly. The packs are applied quickly to minimize the chance of cooling.

It is usually unnecessary to use ointments or oils to protect the skin, but if a patient shows signs of sensitivity to the application or extreme dryness of the skin it is advisable to use some type of oil on the skin.

It should be remembered that during the administration of the hot foments the following points are to be observed.

(*a*) Care should be taken to prevent unnecessary stimulation.
(*b*) The skin should be closely observed for signs of hypersensitiveness.
(*c*) Care should be taken not to set up inimical reflexes.
(*d*) Administer the treatment so as to improve the circulation.
(*e*) Preserve the vitality of the tissue.
(*f*) Gain the patient's confidence by allaying any fear or apprehension.
(*g*) Avoid chilling of the part before, during, or after the treatment.

Procedure in preparation of hot foments:

Requisites:
(*a*) A blanket for under the patient.
(*b*) Soft flannel or woolen blanket material cut in sizes varying according to the areas treated.
(*c*) Oiled silk or thin rubberized sheeting cut in sizes a bit larger than the foments.
(*d*) Flannel or blanket material used as coverings for each hot foment, preferably sewed to the rubberized pieces.

(*e*) Safety pins to secure the pack.
(*f*) Sand bags to stabilize the part after packing.
(*g*) Vaseline or oil for dryness or sensitivity of the skin after packing.

Purpose of Hot Foments:
(*a*) To relieve pain resulting from muscular spasm by aiding in relaxation of the muscle fibers.
(*b*) To stimulate the absorption of exudate, or products of inflammation.
(*c*) To stimulate nerve centers in the skin.
(*d*) To improve the circulation of the part.

Technique:
(*a*) Assemble all material which will be needed.
(*b*) Sort the pieces needed for the particular parts to be treated.
(*c*) Place all pieces to be heated in the machine so that the piece to be used last will be put in the machine first, and the piece to be used first will be put in the machine last, to be on top.
(*d*) Arrange the oiled silk and woolen pieces to be used as coverings under the part to be packed, with the pins close by. These pieces are more easily handled if they are sewed together.
(*e*) Apply the packs to all parts which may be reached from the supine position before turning the patient.
(*f*) Leave the patient resting in a comfortable position.

MUSCLE FUNCTION TESTING

Evaluating Muscle Function Tests.—The importance of accurately measuring muscle strength in the after-care of infantile paralysis is obvious. It is necessary to make a critical evaluation of muscle testing commonly used and endeavor to establish an instrument whereby a standard unit of expression of muscle strength is obtained.

A short review of tests devised in the past shows the unreliability and inaccuracy of most tests. At first charts were developed consisting of anterior and posterior views of the body with an outline of important muscles which were then shaded for various muscle strengths. This did not show whether the partially paralyzed muscles were slightly or severely damaged.

"The Spring Balance Muscle Test" showed a gain or loss in muscular strength, but very weak muscles could not be tested; it also required consistent effort on the part of the patient,

The grading system found most satisfactory was devised by Lovett and tested the strength of muscles as elicited by resistance testing with or against gravity. At the present time there seems to be some unanimity in the use of this method of testing; however, there is a wide diversity of nomenclature and manner of application of the test. For example, the Mayo Clinic uses "O" as the highest grade or symbol for a normal muscle; the Kendalls measure their system of grading on the percentage scale; Legg and Merrill grade the muscles in the same manner as Lovett except that they add the plus and minus signs to provide for greater accuracy in degree of muscle power. This method or a modification of it is commonly used in hospitals today, but most examiners, each hospital, and every technician have a somewhat different interpretation of the grades. The range of motion, the number of times a movement can be performed without causing fatigue, or the amount of manual resistance given by the examiner determine the grade. Although this method of examination is not a mathematically accurate one, it has the advantage of requiring no apparatus and of providing a graded series of tests for estimating muscular power. Its main weakness at the present is the lack of standardization of nomenclature and uniformity of symbols. For example, Kendall lists fourteen grades beginning with "zero" and ending with "normal plus;" Lowman lists ten different grades using numerals from zero to nine. It can readily be seen that there is no uniformity in testing methods or in the terms used. The terms used may not be important in themselves, as long as all individuals in the same institution know their meaning; however, for the sake of students and all who consult literature, the ambiguity and diversity of terms is very confusing. Standardization of nomenclature and symbols, therefore, is highly desirable, with clear definitions included.

Criteria in Evaluating Muscle Function Tests.—It is well recognized in the field of tests and measurements that validity, reliability, and objectivity be kept in mind when evaluating a test. The following are examples:

Validity of Muscle Testing.—A good test must of necessity be designed to measure accurately with each repeated use. For instance, a skilled examiner will carefully select and use consistently, proved testing positions and movements which will be able to isolate muscle action as nearly as it is possible. For this test to be valid, it is desirable for the same operator who makes the first test to carry through on all subsequent tests, using the same methods on later tests.

Reliability.—The accuracy of the test itself concerns not the isolating of muscle action as nearly as possible, but rather the measurement of the strength of the motion itself. Here, the factor of gravity on a part must be considered, as also keeping constant the weight to be moved. This involves the length of the lever arm, whether the arm is extended or flexed at the elbow when being abducted, the position assumed in testing, whether favorable for gravity to aid in the movement, whether the segment is being asked at another time to act against the pull of gravity. Reliability is also influenced by a factor which is not usually considered by individuals administering the test. It is the "sense of gymnastics" with which the patient may or may not be endowed. This innate "sense of spatial relationships" controls the readiness with which various patients may or may not respond to a command to perform a certain movement. Even though two patients may suffer similar residual muscular weaknesses, one may respond quickly to a command, whereas another may require several practice periods before "habit" patterns are established and the proprioceptive neurons in muscle, tendons, and joints inform him of the positional status of the segment. The degree with which a patient may respond to the operator varies with the individuals, as a *personal relationship* is involved which influences the reliability of the test, as also does the variability with which the patient responds, even to the same operator from day to day. As the human equation element also enters into and influences the treatment, it is necessary to maintain good rapport between patient and technician to achieve maximum reliability from the tests.

Objectivity.—In the objective test there is a high degree of uniformity with which various persons may score the same test. If muscle "groups" are graded by careful directions, which have been clearly defined and standardized for each movement, a relatively high degree of objectivity necessarily results.

Standardization of a scheme of muscle evaluation which may be uniformly employed by all physicians and technicians skilfully trained in the technique of one selected method is much to be desired. The grades must be clearly defined and the definitions universally accepted. A testing position for each grade and for each movement must be agreed upon. For instance, in grading the function of a quadriceps muscle, the patient should be placed on his side with the knee flexed, until the muscle is able to function against gravity.

The testing of muscle function is a highly specialized field and anatomical knowledge, although necessary, is not sufficient, as great skill and much experience are required for expert grading of paralyzed or partially paralyzed muscles. It is to be desired that an objective measurement of muscle function be obtained as early as such a test may be carried out with reliable accuracy and without detriment to the patient.

As it takes much skill and practice for accurate testing of muscles, a physician should check them from time to time, although the same technician should be selected for all testing of a particular patient in subsequent trials.

Grading of Muscle Function Tests.—Muscle function may be tested for isolated action and for group muscle movements.

Isolated Muscle Testing.—To test for the isolated action of a muscle is not consistent with a program which involves re-education of the muscles by exercise. It is used principally for diagnostic purposes and is best accomplished with the aid of electrical currents; therefore, will not be considered in a program designed for re-education by therapeutic exercises.

Group Muscle Function Testing.—Since the action of single muscles cannot be isolated accurately by volitional effort, muscle groups are usually graded instead of the individual muscles. This manner of testing is the most practical for use in determining muscle function and is best performed in the early stages under water where gravity, friction, and inertia are eliminated. The testing may be carried out on a highly polished table instead if a Hubbard tank is not available. The method is somewhat the same, although allowance must be made for the effect of gravity.

The determination of the grade depends upon the following factors:

(*a*) Can or cannot a muscle perform against gravity?
(*b*) Can or cannot the friction of the table and the friction of the joint be overcome?
(*c*) How many times may the movement be repeated without causing fatigue? (Indicate by fibrillary twitchings.)
(*d*) Can the muscle perform through the full range of motion normal for it?
(*e*) Is there uniform resistance given by the operator at each testing period?
(*f*) Is the factor of gravity constant?
(*g*) Are the testing positions standardized? (Is the lever arm the same in each repeated movement?)
(*h*) Are all conditions the same in subsequent tests?

A Selected System of Grading for Muscle Function.—A muscle test in the field of functional measurements is the examination by which the capacities of muscles and changes in those capacities are evaluated in terms of amounts, and progress of skill in testing will develop upon a general reception of fundamental units of expression of acceptable symbols and terms.

The system chosen here as a method for interpreting and using the results obtained from the measurement of muscle function of residual paralysis, as elicited by the resistance test with and against gravity, were established as a standard unit of expression of muscle strength by the Committee on Standards of the National Foundation for Infantile Paralysis and recently published in *The Journal of the American Medical Association*, May 5, 1945.

Standardized Graph for Muscle Performance

5 = N	= Normal	=	No apparent deficiency.
4 = G	= Good	=	Approximates normal but fatigues more readily.
3 = F	= Fair	=	Where part can perform function against gravity but is obviously weak.
2 = P	= Poor	=	Where muscle is so weakened that it cannot perform its function against gravity but with the removal of gravity can function.
1 = T	= Trace	=	Where there is slight contractility of the muscle.
0 = O	= Zero	=	No evidence of contractility of muscle fibers.

It is to be hoped that all who are called upon to grade paralyzed or partially paralyzed muscles will make use of the table recommended above and avoid the confusion and ambiguity formerly associated with the terms used in this most important part of the after-care of paralyses.

A Key Graph to be Used in Underwater Testing of Muscle Function in a Hubbard Tank.—The system given below was devised by one of the authors of this book for the purpose of elucidating the finer gradients of muscle function as elicited by underwater testing. It was necessary to give a more detailed chart to avoid errors of judgment and to increase the objectivity of the test itself. As only a real expert in testing can tell, for instance, the difference between a poor minus and a poor plus muscle, it was found that students acquired that skill more rapidly with the aid of a more detailed graph.

Key Graph for Underwater Testing of Muscle Function

N	Normal	=	Normal action of muscles for the particular patient.
G+	Good plus	=	Can take less than normal resistance; muscular weakness.
G	Good	=	Can take graded resistance plus the force of gravity.
G−	Good minus	=	Muscles can move against gravity in any position.

F+	Fair plus	= Muscles can move against gravity if they are in a favorable position, but can take no additional resistance. Range is complete.
F	Fair	= The strength of both antagonists is better balanced, and patient can move parts against the resistance of water plus slightly applied resistance by the operator, but not against gravity.
F−	Fair minus	= Patient can complete the whole arc and can hold position in the water.
P+	Poor plus	= Patient can move the whole segment through the complete arc without assistance, and against the resistance of the water.
P	Poor	= Patient is beginning to be able to move the part but cannot complete the whole arc without assistance.
P−	Poor minus	= There is a well defined contraction. Muscle tone is better, and patient is beginning to help move the segment by initiating the movement.
T+	Trace plus	= There is a well defined and visually observable contraction, but patient cannot move the segment yet.
T	Trace	= Palpable contraction, but muscle tone is hypotonic. Patient cannot move segment.
T−	Trace minus	= Slight palpable contraction, muscle tone is flaccid; no movements.
O	Zero or totally paralyzed	= Muscle completely flaccid.

Charting Muscle Function Tests.—In charting the result of a volitional muscle function test the following graph is used, which has been adopted by the National Foundation for Infantile Paralysis.

Principles of Testing for Muscle Action.—It is our belief that it is possible to obtain a true test for muscle action in the volitional test, scientifically applied. It is the only test which takes into account the two elements of muscular action, the contraction of one muscle and the relaxation of its opponent, the two constituting the true elements of muscular action.

For example, if the leg is bent back at the knee, the flexors of the knee contract and the quadriceps relaxes and elongates with the contraction of the hamstrings. In other words, flexion is not an unregulated action of the flexors, but it is regulated by means of the extensors so that a too forcible action of the benders is prevented. Relaxation then is essentially an active and not a passive state of muscle, and the relaxation of the opponent goes hand in hand with the action of the contracting muscle. With the observation of this fact it has been reasoned that in order to obtain muscular control and useful movement, nerve impulses must be present that can *prevent* muscles from acting. It is in order at this point to digress from our discussion on the volitional testing for muscular action

Muscle Examination

Patient's Name__________ Chart No.__________

Date of Birth__________ Name of Institution__________

Date of Onset__________ Attending Physician __________ M. D.

Diagnosis:

	LEFT								RIGHT	
					Examiner's Initials					
					Date					
NECK					Flexors					NECK
					Extensors					
TRUNK					Flexor					TRUNK
					Extensors — thoracic					
					Extensors — lumbar					
					R. ext. obl. } L. int. obl. } Rotators { L. ext. obl. { R. int. obl.					
					Elevation of pelvis					
HIP					Flexors					HIP
					Extensors					
					Abductor					
					Adductors					
					External Rotators					
					Internal Rotators					
					Sartorius					
					Tensor fasciae latae					
KNEE					Flexor — outer hamstring					KNEE
					Flexors — inner hamstrings					
					Extensors					
ANKLE					Plantar-flexors — Gastroc. & Soleus					ANKLE
					Plantar-flexor — Soleus					
FOOT					Invertor — Anterior tibial					FOOT
					Invertor — Posterior tibial					
					Evertor — Peroneus brevis					
					Evertor — Peroneus longus					
TOES (4 lateral)					Flexors — metatarsophalangeal					TOES (4 lateral)
					Extensors — metatarsophalangeal					
					Flexor — proximal interphalangeal					
					Flexor — distal interphalangeal					
					Abductors					
					Adductors					
HALLUX					Flexor — metatarsophalangeal					HALLUX
					Flexor — interphalangeal					
					Extensor — interphalangeal					

Additional Data:

Face__________

Speech__________

Swallowing__________

Diaphragm__________

Intercostals__________

KEY

100%	5	N	Normal	Complete range of motion against gravity with full resistance.
75%	4	G	Good*	Complete range of motion against gravity with some resistance.
50%	3	F	Fair*	Complete range of motion against gravity.
25%	2	P	Poor*	Complete range of motion with gravity eliminated.
10%	1	T	Trace	Evidence of slight contractility. No joint motion.
0	0	0	Zero	No evidence of contractility.
	S or SS		Spasm	Spasm or severe spasm.
	C or CC		Contracture	Contracture or severe contracture.

*Muscle Spasm or contracture may limit range of motion. A question mark should be placed after the grading of a movement that is incomplete from this cause.

and study the mechanism which involves the reciprocal innervation of muscles spoken of by Sherrington and others.

It is customary to think of a nerve impulse as a form of energy that can cause a muscle to contract, but in order to procure muscular control in movements, the opponents relax progressively to elicit a smooth movement. This is not a passive failure to act on the part of the opponent, but is an actual inhibition with less tone than is present in the normal resting state. It seems necessary for this mechanism to be present for the economical use of muscles, for in

LEFT										RIGHT
					Examiner's Initials					
					Date					
SCAPULA					Abductor — Serratus anterior					SCAPULA
					Adductor — middle trapezius					
					Adductors — Rhomboids					
					Elevators					
					Depressor					
SHOULDER					Flexors					SHOULDER
					Extensors					
					Abductors					
					Horizontal Abductor					
					Horizontal Adductor					
					External rotators					
					Internal rotators					
ELBOW					Flexors					ELBOW
					Extensors					
FOREARM					Supinators					FOREARM
					Pronators					
WRIST					Flexor — radial deviation					WRIST
					Flexor — ulnar deviation					
					Extensors — radial deviation					
					Extensor — ulnar deviation					
FINGERS					Flexors — metacarpophalangeal					FINGERS
					Extensors — metacarpophalangeal.					
					Flexor — proximal interphalangeal					
					Flexor — distal interphalangeal					
					Abductors					
					Adductors					
					Opponens — 5th finger					
THUMB					Opponens					THUMB
					Flexor — metacarpophalangeal					
					Extensor — metacarpophalangeal					
					Flexor — interphalangeal					
					Extensor — interphalangeal					
					Abductors					
					Adductor					
					MEASUREMENTS					
CHEST					Inspiration					CHEST
					Expiration					
ABDOMEN					Umbilicus to Ant. Sup. Spine					ABDOMEN
LOWER EXTREMITY					Circumference — mid calf					LOWER EXTREMITY
					Circumference — mid thigh					
					Ant. Sup. spine to int. malleolus					
					Umbilicus to internal malleolus					

Cannot walk Date__________ Walks with crutches Date__________

Stands Date__________ Walks with canes Date__________

Walks with braces Date__________ Walks unaided Date__________

Walks with corset Date__________ Climbs stairs Date__________

Other Apparatus__________

Scoliosis and other deformities__________

Supplied by The National Foundation for Infantile Paralysis, Inc., 120 Broadway, N. Y. 5, N. Y., Publication No. 60.

Revised March 1946

making a movement, force would be wasted if one were obliged to overcome the tone of the opposing group. This is especially true in a state of excitement when the tone is greatly increased. However, a muscular movement properly performed in which there is inhibition of the opponents is economical, graceful, and useful for definite purposes.

Sherrington, the greatest authority on this topic, describes an experiment in which he uses an animal from which the brain has been removed and whose muscles are, therefore, under the influence alone of the spinal cord and the autonomic neurons. The animal exhibits an extraordinary amount of muscular tone, which in itself indicates that the general influence of the brain is to inhibit the tonic action of muscles. If the flexors of the knee are severed at the origin, but otherwise kept intact and then stimulated by an electric shock, it is found that even though the flexor muscles are severed from the joint, the joint will flex. This is accounted for by the fact that the stimulation of the muscle and its subsequent contraction likewise stimulates the sensory endings in it. A message goes into the spinal cord that causes an inhibition of the tone of the extensors whose tonic action is to hold the joint extended, but on receiving fewer impulses by the inhibitory process, are unable to hold the joint stiff. As soon as the stimulation ceases, the extensors once more retrieve their tone and again the joint is extended.

To account for *reciprocal innervation* we note the effect of stimulation of a motor nerve. All muscles supplied by this nerve will contract, irrespective of their actions, and no purposeful movement is brought about. The motor nerve (isolated) does not contain inhibitory fibers. In reflex action, on the contrary, the muscular response consists of a coördinate movement, as the flexors contract while the extensors automatically relax. Although the mechanism whereby the extensors are inhibited is not fully understood, the inhibitory effect must be developed in the reflex center, at a synapse between the afferent and efferent neurons, for as has just been said, the motor nerves have no inhibitory fibers. We consequently speak of a *central inhibitory state* as well as a *central excitatory state.*

Reciprocal inhibition is also seen in voluntary movement. For example, in flexing the arm at the elbow, the contraction of the brachialis is accompanied by reciprocal inhibition of the triceps; in extending the elbow, the triceps contracts while the brachialis relaxes.

The above principles should of necessity be considered in the scientific application of volitional muscle testing. This is especially true in the executing of a new movement for the first time as, for example, in re-educating muscles in the various paralyses. In order that a new movement be executed for the first time, the pyramidal cells of the brain must come into action, and just as the pyramidal neurons at the beginning of the movement stimulate some motor groups and inhibit others, so the impulses coming in from joints, muscles, and skin influence some muscles to contract and others to relax, each in its turn, and thereby guide the execution of the later phases of the movement. At each stage of the movement these sensory impulses are acting to guide the muscular contractions of the next stage. The new movement becomes reflex as practice continues. In other words, the pyramidal cells or "higher level" nerve mechanism is replaced in control by the "lower level" mechanism, that of muscular sense in particular.

When the individual performs an old and familar movement, he can recognize it by muscular sense; that is, he can tell with his eyes shut whether he is walking or running and where the various parts of his body are at a given moment. This he does by muscular sense or by the sensory impression arising in his joints and muscles. Now these same sensory impulses that give rise to a sense of position, and movement, also guide the performance of reflex acts, but have to be developed by repeated performances of the movement. With practice there is a development of the synapses that are most traversed by impulses in the performance of the movement, with the result that the path thus blazed is ever after easier to follow.

The volitional testing of muscles should accordingly take into account all the principles herein laid out for the re-education of muscles, in that it is essential to understand the inherent power in the muscles and the neuromuscular mechanism to elicit a true performance of the muscle in any accurate test for function.

Aptly applied, the volitional test enables one to determine the minimum action from which the muscle can be re-educated up to the maximum. For still greater accuracy, several factors must also be considered.

1. The ancestral history of the muscle must be considered, including the paths along which it has acquired its maximum function.

2. The effect of gravity must be considered; the placing of the origin and insertion of the muscle as nearly as possible on a level, the avoidance of frictional effects (may use a highly polished board or underwater exercise), the position in which the "movement of force" is greatest (the most favorable position in which the muscle can act), as well as the position in which the leverage can be most effective.

3. A thorough knowledge of the action, origin and insertions of muscles, of course, is quite necessary in making any type of muscle function test.

4. There should be complete normal range of movement of the components of the joint, and should contraction of an opponent

have been allowed to occur through neglect it must at first be overcome by passive stretching before re-education or even testing can accurately take place. Many times a muscle condemned as hopeless is really a recovered one, mechanically prevented from acting because of the shortened condition of the antagonists.

Rules Used in Testing for Muscle Function to be Observed in Testing and Re-education of Muscles.—The same movements applied in muscle testing are used thereafter in re-education of the muscles.

1. Strong muscles are not to be treated at the expense of weak ones.
2. Watch for fatigue and fibrillary twitchings.
3. Prevent deformities by restricting weight bearing movements. Use splinting and braces in prevention of and passive stretching in the releasing of contractures.
4. Prevent the stretching of *weak* or partially paralyzed muscles.
5. Teach the patient mental re-education, or the building of new nerve paths as well as the inhibition of the synergistic action of those muscles which merely aid in the movement by fixing the joint.
6. Avoid passive movements in which the patient does not coöperate. Use assistive movements first.
7. Avoid use of muscles which are weak.
8. Move through a full arc of motion. (There is a difference of opinion concerning this.) The operator should complete the arc when the patient is unable to do so, but the patient should be instructed to concentrate on completing the arc.
9. Apply effort in one direction only.
10. Add resistive movements when patient is able to move the part. This is to strengthen the muscles.
11. Daily treatments are more effective at first.

MUSCLE RE-EDUCATION IN POLIOMYELITIS

The Rôle of the Neuromuscular Mechanism in Re-education.—Physical medicine is to be applied early and continued throughout the average two-year period of convalescence. Before any description of treatment for paralysis it is necessary to study some of the physiological principles affecting re-education.

Disturbed Motion Patterns.—The theory that a non-functioning muscle may result from a physiological and not an organic nerve lesion has long been recognized and used in muscle re-education methods; however, there has been much ambiguity and confusion of descriptive nomenclature. Many expressions such as "neuromuscular estrangement," "forgotten or interrupted nerve paths," "disturbed motion patterns," and "mental alienation" have been used for this condition by as many different authorities on the subject. Furthermore, these terms have been applied to as many different neuromuscular diseases: poliomyelitis, hemiplegia, Bell's palsy, hysterical paralysis, brachial plexus paralysis, traumatic neurosis, as well as post-fracture cases in which the patient has not had occasion to use the part for prolonged periods. In these and many other cases of inability to produce a voluntary, purposeful movement in a muscle in spite of the fact that the nerve paths to it are anatomically intact, muscle re-education, based on the theory that this is a physiological block and should be distinguished from the organic interruption resulting from destruction of a motor neuron, is found profitable. Muscle re-education will of necessity call into use the higher centers as in the performance of a "new act," thereby re-establishing by practice the motion paths necessary for the movement.

Obviously the same measures also may be used profitably where there has been an "organic" break in the nerve fiber without destruction of the nerve cell, provided there is a possibility of its regeneration.

Disturbance in the neuromuscular motion patterns in poliomyelitis may be produced in several ways:

1. A muscle is pulled beyond its normal resting length by its opponent which may be in spasm.
2. A muscle may become estranged when pain is produced in its involved opponent by an attempt of the unaffected muscle to contract.
3. The spasm, or its later results, in an affected muscle may be so severe that the "braking" action or check on the normal opposing muscle may discourage the latter enough to produce a blocking of impulses to the muscle.
4. The disease may produce changes in the nervous system which do not actually harm the cells or fibers but do cause loss of conduction power and interference with normal neuromuscular function.

Neuromuscular Imbalance.—The asynchronous action between muscular opponents, or even within a muscle itself, may be attributable to either one of the two following conditions:

1. Diffusion of impulses as a result of the spreading of motor impulses intended for a certain muscle to other muscles or groups of muscles, because of conditions of pain on attempted motion of an involved muscle which is unable to perform.

2. A spreading of impulses occurring within the involved muscle itself so that ineffective contraction is produced instead of a coordinated rhythmic contraction producing maximum motion.

Functional Ability of Muscles as Determined by Positional Factors.—*Group 1:* Muscles which contract within their normal resting length, as the gastrocnemius.

Group 2: Muscles which have to be removed from their normal resting length before a suitable contraction can occur to perform the primary action of the muscle; as the quadriceps to extend the knee.

Group 3: Muscle groups with separate origin and common insertion and multiple actions, as the biceps of the arm.

Group 4: Muscle grouns with dual origins and insertions and muscle actions, as the hamstrings of the thigh.

Group 5: Muscles which stabilize certain structural positions to permit the primary action of other muscle groups, as trapezius in the shoulder girdle.

The last group is important in that it has been found that when synergists or fixers of a part (the shoulder or pelvis) are allowed to take over the action of the prime mover, it is impossible to re-educate the muscle which should normally perform this movement. It is found that if the former group is taught to exercise its own original function (that of fixing the joint) then the group which is being taught to perform its prime movement has a better chance to complete the movement in a normal manner.

Summary of Principles for Muscle Testing and Re-education.—*First Principle.*—An enfeebled muscle cannot contract unless and until its antagonist relaxes in comformity.

Second Principle.—The second principle is to make sure that the patient's muscles at least know how to perform the prescribed movement and that he realizes fully what is desired.

Third Principle.—The muscle should be required to perform no work that is impossible for it to do. An enfeebled muscle will not even make an attempt to do that which it knows to be impossible for it. The result is that the antagonists are thrown into a condition of firm contraction; as for instance, if the abductors are incapable of raising the arm, the adductors contract so as to do their best to assist the elevation of the arm by means of scapular movement. Synergistic action is called upon to perform the movement in an incoördinated effort to procure the motion. To counteract this the therapist must insure that only two muscle groups act within the limb, the muscle he wishes to be contracted and the antagonists which must reciprocally relax.

Fourth Principle.—The fourth principle is to graduate activity so that, when one feat has been accomplished, a second shall be devised which, in its performance, will entail an almost imperceptible, but none the less real, increased expenditure of energy.

Fifth Principle.—This principle involves the rôle of the synergist in the contemplated act. Thus, when the patient performs a certain movement, it seems quite possible that this particular effort is performed in the main by some one muscle while others may give subsidiary aid and act as synergists. Therefore, when performing some particular movement, one of those synergists may assume the primary rôle while the normal prime mover of the act assumes that of the synergist. However, with a lack of the knowledge of synergistic action, it is rather difficult for the operator to comply with the fifth principle in muscle training, that of always selecting as the first movement in training the muscle the one action which in normal life represents the sole and true function of the particular muscle to be re-educated.

Sixth Principle.—The sixth principle entails a personal element in training that can be developed only with experience. It consists of the blending of rest and activity. Few conditions will retard the progress of muscle recovery as quickly as fatigue produced in the muscle from overactivity. Maximal effort should be employed with caution, usually not more than once during each exercise period.

Seventh Principle.—This principle concerns the range of movement or arc through which the muscle may be carried. The muscle should be taught to contract and perform as much of the arc as it is possible; then the rest of the range of movement should be carried out for the patient, so that complete nerve paths may be established without fatiguing the muscle.

Eighth Principle.—This well-known and recognized principle holds that no enfeebled muscle must ever be stretched.

Ninth Principle.—It is well to recognize the signs of having overexercised a part. If on any day the power of contraction or the amount of movement is less than usual, all voluntary effort at movement that day should be postponed.

Tenth Principle.—This is one of the most important principles to consider in treating any case of paralysis. It is the position to be assumed by the patient between times appointed for definite exercise. The use of splints and posterior half shells for rest of the quadriceps when needed is much to be urged. Proper instruction of the patient in this matter may make the difference between recovery and deformity.

Eleventh Principle.—This principle requires that there is no need to check all movement of the antagonists, whereby some coördination in the task of re-educating may be lost. Though it is imperative that there should be no overdevelopment of the antagonist at the expense of the enfeebled muscle, it is necessary to limit its activity only to the point that the weakened muscle is not stretched.

Twelfth Principle.—The fullest activity of all uninjured muscles in the limb should be encouraged so that there may be maintained an improved circulation to the parts keeping intact the nutrition and the joint and muscle sense against the day of recovery when the better part of the burden of weight may be cast on the unaffected member. Disuse atrophy is often harder to cure than atrophy resulting from nerve injury. The one precaution which should be taken is that all measures to prevent stretching of the enfeebled muscle should be considered.

Application of Muscle Re-education in Poliomyelitis.—Some of the conditions below are due to the disturbed physiology of the neuromuscular mechanism in poliomyelitis.

Pain is an important symptom, causing spasm in certain muscle groups and a persistent weakness of the opponent on account of paralysis, partial or complete; the weakness may be due to the shortened spastic state of the antagonist. In many cases this may be the cause for the speedy recovery of some muscles when the spasm is released in an opponent in accordance with the law of reciprocal innervation, or unequal distribution of nerve stimuli.

Another mechanism which may account for delayed function is the adaptation of muscles to joint positions occurring because of positional stimuli from the proprioceptive reflexes of muscle, joints, and ligaments. In this condition the afferent or sensory nerves are always intact, but the efferent or motor nerves are disturbed on account of the pathology of the cell in the anterior horn; consequently, the muscles are unable to move a joint segment although the sensory impulses arising in the muscle, joint, and ligament are intact.

When muscle function is retarded by the action of the synergists performing as substitutes for the prime mover, there is a misdirection of nerve impulse to the region which may take several forms. The opposing muscle may contract, or unrelated muscles try to act; for example, a muscle which usually aids in the movement by fixing a joint may try to perform the prime movement. Yet another form of substitution may result in a misdirection of nerve impulses within the muscle itself, as in the case of a good sternocleidomastoid being unable to flex the head because it is trying to raise the rib cage. The patient is usually unaware of substitution which leads to the development of a condition of muscular imbalance.

Muscular imbalance is the result of a misdirection of impulses because of a disorganization of motor impulses at the site of the lesion, and is not to be confused with substitution. There is increasingly less tendency toward substitution or asynchronization if the patient visualizes the movement in his higher centers. If the muscles do respond during the convalescent period, the paralysis may have been due to temporarily lost reflex patterns.

The physiological blocking of impulses is a condition occurring in the opposing muscles of those in spasm. These opposing muscles are occasionally non-functioning not because they are paralyzed from the destruction of the anterior horn cells, but because for some more or less undetermined reason the impulse is unable to reach that particular muscle, even though the nerve path to it is intact. It may be considered the divorcement of the muscle or muscles from the brain as a result of a physiological block. Some of the possible causes of mental estrangement of muscles may be as follows:

1. As a muscle goes into spasm, it pulls its opponent from its normal resting length and hinders it from a normal contraction by removing it from the position in which it can best do so.

2. The spasm may be so severe that it acts as an effectual "brake" on the opposing muscle.

3. The opponent may be estranged to prevent any stretching of the tight painful muscles in spasm.

4. The virus may cause a disruption in the whole nervous system which interferes with normal neuromuscular action.

Muscles cut off from the higher centers and not re-educated become permanently non-functioning.

In the treatment of muscles which have lost established reflex patterns an endeavor to eliminate spasm in the opposing group should be begun immediately, and then re-education processes may be started, using the following aids in the process:

1. The establishment of new motion patterns is aided by the stimulation of muscles through light scratching or by drawing the finger across the site of insertion of the muscle which is expected to make the movement. This creates proprioceptive reflex action and aids in overcoming the physiologically interrupted motor path by drawing the patient's attention to the site of motion.

Another mechanism which should be used is to have the patient picture the movement with eyes closed, concentrating on the movement while the operator performs it for him directly after stimulating the muscle at its tendon. The patient should make a conscientious effort to help in the movement also. This process helps in the establishment of a new reflex for the motion and leads to the restoration of function ultimately, if the muscles are non-functioning as the result of a loss of neuromuscular habit patterns.

2. The elimination of spasm is of primary importance, as a spasm results from a series of involuntary contractions and may progress from spasm to a physiological shortening, and even on to an organized contracture, if it is not released before that time.

There are three stages of spasm, the first of which constitutes an acute involuntary contraction with hypertonicity being constant, as well as pain and an exaggerated tonus. The muscle is hyperirritable in this acute stage. In the second stage, there is an involuntary shortening, a hypertonic condition, and while there may still be some pain, there is no longer an exaggerated tonus. In the third or contracture state, there is usually little or no pain, and no exaggerated tonus, but the muscle has become permanently shortened and if untreated, it continues in that state and creates a deformity.

The time in which a spasm results in a permanent contracture is varied but may take from six weeks to six months. A muscle which has become shortened if it is in the back may cause a scoliosis because of the short muscle groups on the side of the concavity of the spinal curve and the elongated groups on the convexity side. A strong inelastic muscle will not allow bone growth in the young because the epiphysis cannot exert enough pressure to lengthen the muscles.

3. After the painful inflammatory period has passed, the spastic groups are stretched passively every day during the treatment periods and the patient is given those exercises which he is capable of performing and which will tend to keep the tight groups on a sustained stretch.

Muscle re-education necessarily is ineffectual if the opposing muscle group is shortened because of spasm.

Theory of Underwater Gymnastics and Table Exercises in Muscle Re-education.—Fundamental exercises in water (90° to 93°F.) influence the muscle groups most vital to the development of swimming skill and have a desirable effect on the anti-gravity muscles, whose tonicity is so important in the maintenance of good alignment in the erect posture. The exercises used in a Hubbard tank must of necessity differ from those which may be given in a pool, because of the limitation of space and depth. However, any muscle group in the body may be re-educated within the confines of the tank.

The first excursion into the tank should be one of orientation for the patient so that he may lose any possible fear of the water, and learn what is expected of him, for his coöperation is of the utmost importance. After the topographical inspection and muscle function test, a plan for the particular set of exercises required by the patient is formulated. A preliminary detailed examination of the individual's muscles is essential in the prescription for exercises to be given a patient with poliomyelitis.

The exercises follow through in a manner similar to the movement given at the time of the muscle function test; however, the movements are graded to the degree of ability of the muscles which are to perform. For example, most of the exercises given to very weak or flaccid muscles are assistive to the extent that from the very first the patient is asked to coöperate mentally by closing his eyes and formulating a mental picture of the movement which is about to take place. At the same time, the operator stimulates the muscle at its point of insertion, so as to direct the flow of impulses to the proper area. Then the operator moves the segment while the patient is urged to "get a pull" from the muscle.

We believe that the segment should be moved through the full arc always, so as to obtain a complete mental picture of the movement. However, most of the movement is probably done at first by the operator to prevent fatiguing the muscles. With consistent effort the patient is found to be helping more and more in the movement and in the process of time is able to make the complete arc by himself. As the muscle gains in function and strength, graded resistance is steadily added. Later when the patient can do the whole movement and take some resistance in the water, he is placed on table exercises to be given alternately with the water exercises. A muscle usually is classified as fair, before table exercises are added.

In the beginning of the re-education process it is noted that the patient makes an endeavor to use the synergists to perform the action of the prime mover when that muscle is flaccid. The patient is discouraged from these movements from the very start and is instructed to send inhibitory impulses to those muscles which try to take over the movement. He may be asked to use each muscle for its own particular function as in re-educating the shoulder abductors the shoulder "fixers" or synergists are put to work in "fixing the shoulder," so that the scapula does not rotate upward in an effort to help raise the arm. After the shoulder is "fixed," the deltoid and supraspinatus are stimulated to attempt the arm abduction movement, and the operator assists by helping raise the arm sideways to shoulder level. When the patient learns to "fix" the shoulder before attempting abduction, it is found that he no longer rotates the whole shoulder to raise the arm. At this point real re-education may be carried out on the "flail" abductor muscles.

If there are contractures or shortened adductor muscles, the arm may be placed in an abduction splint when the patient is not taking exercises. The maintenance of good shoulder position during exercise and muscle rest in the "zero" or neutral position between exercises are factors which greatly speed the recovery of the shoulder abductors.

Frequently, the biceps are in a spastic condition and interfere with flexing the arm in a normal manner. Re-education of weak or paralyzed arm flexors is impossible if the biceps tend to take over the movement with the arm in an unnatural position of supination, giving the patient a "grotesque" appearance. It is found that by re-educating the coracobrachialis to flex the whole arm, and the brachialis the forearm—with the biceps put to rest by keeping the forearm in a pronated position while the arm is moved—the patient is ultimately found to regain the use of both the brachialis and coracobrachialis muscles in a normal manner.

Similar examples are to be found in the lower extremity, where the hip rotators tend to perform adduction when the latter muscles are paralyzed. The patient is instructed here, as in the case just cited (of re-educating the upper extremity), to "fix" the hips before attempting any leg motion. In doing this he simultaneously strengthens the abdominals and prevents synergistic action. When the patient is ready later for walking re-education, it is found that he does not "hitch" his hips in order to swing his leg forward or inward. With hips held firmly and the abdominals firm, he walks in a normal fashion.

In the early stages during exercise periods the patient's legs are placed in half-shell casts for rest of the quadriceps and the foot flexors if they are weak or paralyzed. The casts are made slightly inverted for protection of the muscles which support the long arch.

The back is watched carefully for indications of scoliosis. Exercises are given to stretch the side in spasm and to increase the use of those muscles on the opposite side which are elongated. These are accomplished by lateral bending, flexion and extension exercises to be practiced at regular intervals both in the water and in bed. The abdominal and the erector spinæ muscles are concerned in lateral bending, with both the lower extremities and the pelvis fixed in the exercises given. The exercises are given with the patient lying on the side opposite the affected area. When the patient is prone or recumbent and the pelvis is fixed, lateral bending may be attempted. In the same position abduction of the extended extremity may distinguish a difference in muscle strength between quadratus lumborum and the other lateral abdominal muscles.

CHAPTER X

SPASTIC PARALYSIS

(Synonyms: Little's Disease, Cerebral Palsy)

ETIOLOGY OF SPASTIC PARALYSIS

Causes of the Disease.—One of the most frequent causes of spastic paralysis is an intracranial hemorrhage in the new-born as the result of either birth injuries or a prothrombin deficiency in the infant, especially during the first five days of life. When vitamin K analogues are administered, symptoms of hemorrhage are relieved rapidly. The symptoms are found to be infrequent when the mother is treated with vitamin K previous to childbirth.

Later diseases of infancy such as encephalitis and meningitis may produce spastic symptoms in the child.

Other causes of upper motor paralysis or "cerebral palsy" may be due to the following conditions:

(*a*) Fractures of the spine with the crushing of the cord.

(*b*) Acute knuckles on the spine from tuberculosis.

(*c*) Tumors of the spine penetrating the cord.

(*d*) Spastic (senile) paralysis of the aged, common because of degenerative processes within the cerebral cortex and associated with arteriosclerosis of the brain.

Pathology of Cerebral Palsy.—The pathological findings consist of a general atrophy of the brain with shrinkage and sclerosis of the convolutions, or localized areas of softening and degeneration. The atrophied cortex shows an absence of ganglion cells and nerve fibers, the nerve tissue being replaced by gliosis. There is a loss of control by the brain cortex rather than a loss of power (as in flaccidity from damage of the lower motor cells). The affected muscles are in a tonic or contracted state and the extremities are held stiff and resist passive movements. Tendon reflexes are increased; the Babinski and Oppenheim tests are positive.

Spastic paralysis is present at birth or appears soon afterwards and tends to improve as the child grows older. The new-born babe having the foregoing conditions in the brain shows the following symptoms: convulsions following a difficult resuscitation, and rigidity. Later, digestion is impaired, he has trouble in nursing, and is very restless. He may not sit, talk, or walk at the normal age, and later shows backward tendencies, particularly in his studies.

This is not always the rule, however, as some spastics are bright and quick in certain fields while retarded in others. Occasionally one finds a stricken child who is normally alert and intelligent. The intelligence is directly proportional to the extent of the brain lesion.

Types of Spastic Paralysis.—The general pattern of spasticity depends on the extent of the damage to the motor area of the brain and the extent of the lesion. The type of paralysis affecting one side of the body alone is referred to as a hemiplegia; a paralysis affecting both legs is paraplegia; that affecting both arms and like parts on either side of the body is bilateral paralysis; and the paralysis affecting muscles and joints which are supplied by the damaged area in the brain and have lost their relationship to each other and to other parts of the body is called the athetoid type. In this form of spasticity the muscles and joints perform independently in a wild fashion with uncontrolled, incoördinating movements.

Clinical Findings.—In the general clinical picture of Little's disease there is a paralysis as far as voluntary movement is concerned, but not for reflex (unconscious) movements, for these originate in the cord and medulla. Likewise, as higher centers of the brain (their precise location is unknown) exert an inhibitory influence in muscle tone, a lesion in the corticospinal tract permits the impulses to flow undisturbed and results in exaggerated tonic contraction of the muscles.

The contractures may pull the limbs in positions of deformity. The flexor groups are commonly in a state of hypertonicity, the hamstrings hold the thigh in flexion, and the calf muscles pull the feet in a "tip toe" position. The adductors are also tight and give rise to a characteristic "scissors" gait. The spasticity of the child is increased by any attempt to use the extremities, but he is relaxed during sleep.

There is no atrophy of the muscles, because the circulation is unimpaired. This is due to the fact that circulation to the muscles is controlled by the motor neurons of the lower motor anterior horn of the cord, these nerves being unaffected in the paralysis.

GUIDANCE AND MEDICAL TREATMENT

Psychological Concept in Treatment.—All training should be under a competent neurologist or orthopedic surgeon. The nurse or attendant who undertakes the training of a spastic child must have the hope and faith that with constant effort and patience the child will one day be able to handle himself with expedience.

This hope must be transferred from the attendant to the child so that he will develop a helpful mental attitude and will be incited to exert his best efforts to attain this goal. As the destroyed brain cells do not have the power of regeneration, their function is lost. Thus it remains for other portions of the brain to be re-educated to assume the duties of the lost areas. Because the normal child develops mentally as he acquires motor skill, the spastic child may sometimes be underrated mentally, as he is handicapped in expressing his sensory ideas by movements. Therefore, the improvement of his physical disability through training or surgery explains the concurrent mental gain. In the most severe cases mentality is lacking; these children are hopeless idiots, dribbling saliva, having expressionless faces and small, underdeveloped heads. In milder cases, however, where the lesion is not so great, there is the possibility of restoring the child to some degree of normality.

Muscular Plight.—When the child is an athetoid, the extremities may be in a state of *constant movement.* In the condition of general muscular spasticity where voluntary control is lost, the more powerful muscle groups overcome their weaker antagonists, draw the limbs into a position of deformity, and prevent walking. Thus the spastic child presents to us a picture of muscular imbalance.

It is apparent that if certain areas of the brain are damaged, the muscles supplied by nerves coming from these areas will be abnormal and as a result contractures exist. As more impulses are going to one group than to its antagonistic group, the muscles are out of balance.

Depending on the extent of the brain lesion, one or more limbs may be involved, or all the muscles of the body may be included. Likewise, muscles and joints supplied by the damaged area lose their relation to other parts of the body and perform independently and asynchronously. As the rigid groups do not relax when the antagonistic groups begin to work, the child finds great difficulty in performing any motor activity. This muscular imbalance causes the strained muscles to become soon fatigued.

An all-important factor, not to be overlooked in the rehabilitation process of the spastic child, is a psychologist who has had special training in this field. The spastic child presents an easily ruffled, unstable mental attitude, is either depressed or highly exhilarated, and is more likely than not to meet obstacles with a display of temper. This problem understood by an alert psychologist can perhaps be improved and probably overcome. The experienced psychologist can attain a degree of understanding of the intelligence rating, motor ability, personality traits, and interests of the patient which will enable him to study the child's personal preferences, desires, and ambitions.

Guided by the psychologist, the potentiality of other departments (occupational therapy, physical therapy, and special curriculum) can be greatly increased, procuring results far surpassing ordinary expectations.

Prognosis.—The prognosis should be cautiously derived, as restoration of function depends upon the extent of the central lesion. Gradual spontaneous improvement is to be expected except in those with marked mental deficiency. In milder cases normal function may sometimes be obtained by the proper treatment, and even in the more severe ones there may be improvement.

Medical Treatment.—Medicinal treatment, including the administration of glandular products such as pituitary and thyroid extracts, is of value only in relieving the child of any additional physical burden. Some have faulty diet habits, and disorders of digestion and elimination. These patients should be under the care of a medical consultant.

Operative procedure should not be looked upon as a cure-all for spastic conditions, although it has a prominent place in the rehabilitation process. Not all operations have been found profitable, especially the muscle transplants. Tenotomies and plastic lengthenings of tendons are somewhat more satisfactory than neurectomies. Ramisectomies, favored in the past, have been proved of little value. Tenotomies of the adductor muscles of the thigh, and neurectomy of the obturator nerve for overactive adductors and scissors gait are time-honored procedures. Before any operation is a success there must be certain prerequisites: the child must have gained some sort of balance, his condition must be subject to improvement, and the extent of the brain lesion must be small enough for him to have sufficient intelligence to use with advantage any beneficial effects gained.

Operative Procedures on Central Nervous System.—Sectioning of the sensory nerve root within the spinal canal as they emerge from the cord has been abandoned because of the high mortality rate.

Sympathetic ramisection aims at removal of the immodulated nerve impulses sent out from the cerebellar centers to the peripheral nerves and muscles through the sympathetic nerve fiber. This operation, still in the experimental stage, is quite radical; the results do not justify its use generally.

Operative Procedures on Peripheral Nerves.—The Stoeffel operation is the cutting of a part of the nerve supply to a group of contracted muscles.

10

Nerve resection is based upon the principle that a muscle may be weakened to any desired extent by dividing all or part of its motor nerve supply in order to equalize its strength with that of its antagonist and prevent spasmodic deformities. The nerves usually resected are branches of the obturator, thus weakening the adductor group; branches of the sciatic, thus weakening the hamstring group; branches of the tibial, thus weakening the calf muscles; branches of the median, thus weakening pronator radii teres and flexor muscles of wrist and fingers. This operation, though technically somewhat difficult, is attended by very little surgical risk. The ideal age is about five years, though adults may also be benefited.

Operative Procedures on Tendons and Muscles.—Myotomies and tenotomies are sometimes followed by recurrence because the excessive nervous stimuli are not controlled. The lower attachments of the hamstring group may be detached and transplanted to a forward position into the knee-cap. This weakens the overactive muscles on the back of the thigh and also adds power to the quadriceps. Muscles around the forearm and wrist are also frequently transplanted to advantage.

Mechanical Helps.—If the spastic child is to be fully benefited, all available methods for his rehabilitation should be employed. This includes the use of bracing as well as surgery. Not to be overlooked is the very important rôle that corrective shoes play in gaining better foot mechanics. By "corrective shoes" is meant the building up of the soles and heels on one side or the other by wedge-shaped insertions.

Bracing has a very definite place in the stretching of contractures, and also in holding the joint steady in order to decrease the number of vicarious moves. With this support the child is able to focus his attention on establishing a better balance in learning to walk. The braces should be discarded at the earliest possible time to prevent the child from becoming too dependent on them.

Treatment of Spastic Paralysis by Physical Medicine.—Importance of Relaxation.—When the spastic child enters upon his muscle and gait training, half the battle is won if the technician can induce relaxation. Herein lies the secret of training the extremities toward better coördination function. It takes all the ingenuity, resourcefulness, and patience the technician can summon to his aid to teach the patient to do simple automatic things without becoming tense and excited. In this instance, rhythm plays an important part and the patient relaxes appreciably when a certain pattern is established. By counting or repeating the movement over and over until the motor pattern creates new nerve paths in the brain, the child is taught to inhibit those muscles not necessary, and to use in a deliberate fashion only those normally needed for a special act. Before starting the exercise he must be as relaxed as possible. As the word "relax" probably means nothing to him, the operator can suggest other more meaningful expressions like "feel loose," "feel heavy," "let yourself go." When he learns to lie relaxed, the next step is to teach him to sit in a relaxed position. He should sit squarely with arms straight, hands resting on thighs, the legs slightly apart to overcome the strong adductor muscles, and the feet flat on the floor.

Stretching of Shortened Muscles.—As contractures are the outstanding muscular defect, the first exercises must stretch those shortened groups before any great degree of success in coördination and motor skill is possible. Stretching of the muscles of the entire body may be accomplished by using a machine called the "articulator." Its curative quality is best demonstrated in its use as an adjunct in the treatment of abnormal contractions by the mechanical means of a repeated, rhythmic, sustained stroke of elongation.

Because the very act of stretching a muscle induces relaxation, this type of machine with its slow measured pulls performs this feat very well. The muscles in a relaxed state can be stretched to a greater degree than is otherwise possible.

Exercises for the lower extremities to give the child greater degrees of abduction and external rotation of the thighs, extension of the knees, and dorsiflexion of the feet are requisite. Those for the upper extremities should develop abduction and outward rotation of the shoulder, extension of the elbow and wrist, and extension of the fingers.

It is best to have the first exercises done passively by the technician, as any effort on the part of the patient immediately throws the extremities into incoördinated movements.

Some of the exercises for the thighs follows:

1. Patient lies on back relaxed. Press down on both knees slowly and firmly. Hold the position as long as possible, but do not fatigue muscles.
2. Same position. Roll thighs away from each other and hold as many counts as possible.
3. Same position. Hold foot in dorsiflexion with the knee straight, raise leg as high as possible and hold for a brief time. Repeat with other leg.
4. Same position. Patient moves legs apart in abduction, the technician resisting the movement and bringing them back to midline passively. They should be brought back passively in order to prevent the overactive adductors from working.
5. Patient lying on abdomen. Have him contract the gluteii

while the technician raises the straightened leg upward, supporting it there a few minutes. Repeat with other leg.

6. Patient sits with legs hanging from a table. The technician holds one leg in place and pulls the other away as far as possible, passively bringing the leg back. Repeat with the other leg.

7. Because of shortened heel cords the child must be given exercises which will emphasize dorsiflexion.. The patient sits with feet resting on a stool. The operator, while holding the heel in place, dorsiflexes the foot describing a half circle outward. He holds the foot in this position briefly and releases it quickly. Repeat the exercise with the other foot. Next the patient in the same position with the heels on the stool tries to duplicate the exercise. The downward motion is not to be emphasized. This exercise is for the spastic child who toes in and should be used in conjunction with walking exercises in which he is instructed to swing the heels in as far as possible.

8. An exercise for the head and trunk is given here for the child with poor sitting posture. If the head and body tilt forward, have the child reach for something held over his head enough to make him stretch his arms while the technician supports his back. The body grasped firmly with both hands, he tells the child to push up slowly. These exercises must be repeated over and over again for success.

9. In an exercise to loosen the shoulder, the technician seats the patient in a sitting position, holds the shoulder with one hand and gently rotates the upper arm describing a small circle. This exercise can also be done with patient supine by swinging the arm slowly and gently from the side to the shoulder level. This should be repeated several times but not beyond the point of fatigue.

10. To straighten the elbow, the technician grasps the elbow in one hand in order to steady it, then slowly, gently straightens the child's arm, then brings the hand back up to the shoulder passively and repeats.

11. In relaxing the wrist, the patient's hand is between those of the operator who gently but firmly straightens the wrist and holds the extended position. This is repeated with care not to fatigue the hand.

12. To stretch the forearm, the technician holds the child's elbow in one hand and grasps the child's hand in the other, gently supinating and pronating the hand. It is wise to keep the elbow close to the body and not twist the wrist but rather move the whole length of the forearm.

All the exercises given above may be repeated actively by the patient, the technician offering resistance to the extensor groups and passive motion to the flexors.

Active Exercise to Induce Balance.—After the child has attained enough relaxation and muscle control, the next step is to get him to stand alone. He should stand supported with feet slightly apart and must know that he has the aid of the technician in order that he may have maximum relaxation and feel assured. He should not look down at his feet, and should try to let his arms hang easily at his side. The technician should withdraw his assistance very gradually so that the child will have the feeling of coöperation during his first trials. Later he must be made to feel that he has the power within himself to maintain his balance. All possible encouragement should be given him. When the child is able to stand alone he should then be urged to take a step or two. As a spastic child has a tendency to lift his feet high off the floor, it must be stressed that he should place the heel down first. He should be warned to walk slowly and place all the weight on the forward foot before taking the next step.

Rhythm may be introduced at this point to help establish a better balance. The child can be taught to do a simple balance step by grasping a stall bar; later, releasing his hold for a short time, he will find the beginning steps less fearsome.

As he progresses from the balance step to walking unaided, more active exercises are in order. The child holds to a stall bar and describes a circle with each foot in turn to slow rhythmical counting. Even humming slowly will cause him to make more deliberate movements and prevent him from hurrying through his exercises, though he prefers top speed.

In another exercise he slowly swings his arms in time to music. Later he sways the upper part of his trunk from side to side.

If it is possible to have several children present, they can play rhythm games. The games should be chanted or sung slowly but with definite measures. Some of the old games for groups are "In and out the window," "This is the way we go to church," and "Ring around the Rosie." Marching slowly, swinging arms in time to music is effective. Singing the words to the song as they march is efficacious for speech training.

Because the teaching of rhythm takes an increasingly important place in the training of spastic children, it should be highly regarded by operators in an endeavor to establish balance.

Exercises to Coördinate Mind and Body.—Besides instructing in relaxation, physical therapy also endeavors to teach spastic children coördination. By having certain selected exercises, the child acquires skill and grace in performing definite movements with hands and feet.

The child must be taught first to think the movement out, to relax voluntarily the tight muscle group, and then to contract the opposing group. He must not do this with all the force he can, but should limit the power to just enough to accomplish the desired movement with ease. This difficult task requires great perseverance on the part of both the technician and the patient.

With repeated efforts, in time the child should be able to perform intricate movements with the feet and skilled acts with the hands.

Diversified Exercises for the Spastic.—A few of the exercises helpful in acquiring coördination are given here. Some of the best of these exercises are done with the aid of a Swedish stall bar.

1. The patient slowly climbs up and down the stall bar. As this engages the hands and feet at the same time, it coördinates both extremities.
2. From simple climbing up and down may be evolved more intricate exercises as climbing across from the lower right to the upper left corner.
3. Another version is that of climbing alternate bars.
4. If the patient has enough power in his hands, he can hang by them and perform exercises with the legs.
5. By clinging to the stall bar the patient may do various foot-placing exercises. This is excellent in the backward placing of the foot, as it is hard for a spastic to move his foot in that direction.
6. Ask the child to point to various colored tags hung on different bars with a wand as the colors are called out.
7. The child may try to kick a ball suspended by a string, to induce a definite coördinated movement of the lower extremities.
8. For the smaller spastic child "Pat-a-cake," "Fly Away Birdie," "Three Blind Mice," "Church and Steeple" and "Little Pigs" are excellent for the hands and arms.

Balls are good after the child has learned to grasp them and is able to throw them in a given direction. It is not advisable to begin with them as the child may be discouraged after a few futile efforts.

Tops are suitable for the turning-up movement of the right hand in the older and stronger child. The sort of top designated has an upper part which must be placed on a lower one. The lower part is held in one hand and the upper part wound to the right by the handicapped arm. The strongest finger of the hand releases the lower part down for the spin. There are many other exercises of this kind that a clever technician can employ to effect coördination by enlisting the child's coöperation through play.

Occupational Therapy.—As there is no pleasure more satisfying than that of creating an article with the hands, the spastic child will find diversified amusements as well as a profitable gain in coördination by the training given him in occupational therapy. He should be comfortably placed in a chair low enough to place his feet flat on the floor. If unable to sit up alone, he should be supported in a semi-upright position with his feet placed on a stool. Starting with simple projects, he is advanced as fast as his ability permits to more complicated ones.

When the child's ability is tested, if it is shown that he cannot master a particular problem, his failure should be minimized and a simpler problem selected until he has advanced far enough to overcome the difficult problem. Unfair competition between children should be avoided.

Recreational Therapy for Coördination.—The toys and games given a child should be chosen with a definite purpose. Recommended are those which require the use of both hands, are easily manipulated, exercise certain defective muscle groups correctly, and give the child pleasure and satisfaction when mastered with resulting confidence. With suitable toys available for play he will gain greatly in coördination through exercise.

Suitable toys requiring the use of both hands are the simple ones which follow:

1. Musical dinner gong
2. Magnetic toys
3. Paper and crayons
4. Picture books to color
5. Paper and blunt scissors
6. Sand box
7. Clothes pins to fasten together to make different designs
8. Blocks
9. Boards with pegs and hammer to knock the pegs in
10. Toy piano
11. Bead numerical frames
12. Two-piece tops
13. The ring and post game

One of the simpler forms of play which teaches coördination of the hands is the common block. The child should be taught first how to grasp the block in his hand. After he can hold the block in his hand, he should attempt to place the block in a different place or on top of another block. This gives excellent extension and flexion of the fingers, produces purposeful movements of the upper extremities, and stimulates individual finger work.

Another good form of play having the desired effect of exercising the forearm is the ring and post game. With one hand the child removes the ring from a post held by the other hand and places it on a second post. This is useful in giving extension and flexion of the wrist, raises the shoulder, and relaxes the fingers when the ring drops over the post.

Construction toys are composed of irregularly shaped pieces of wood which have small holes drilled through them. The child fashions different articles by fastening together the bits of wood with bolts which he inserts through the holes and tightens with a nut. This is essentially a coördinated exercise, as both the brain and hands are required to fashion an article from the parts.

For a small child the little toy carpenter sets are of much value. He learns to use the hammer with the instructor's aid. Later when he acquires sufficient control, he can bring the hammer in contact with a rather large head of a small nail. It does not take long for the child to learn to hit the nail head. Next he learns to use the claw-hammer for pulling out the nails, an operation requiring two hands. Later he may master the use of a small hack saw and begin to construct small articles.

Another useful instrument is the jig saw. This exercise can be given enabling the child to cut out small and intricate pieces of wood with the jig saw. This gives hip flexion and extension, knee flexion and extension, and coördination of hands and feet.

One of the most definitely profitable experiences a child may have results from learning to weave and braid. These exercises give good coördination for both hands as well as exercises involving individual fingers, wrists, elbows, and the entire arms and shoulders. Weaving satisfies an innate desire to create, and at the same time effects upper extremity control and coördination. There is a bedside loom which can be clamped to a table. It can be handled by a small child, the fingers doing the shifting of the shed instead of the feet as on a larger loom. Many things can be made on this type of loom—purses, scarfs, runners, etc.

In most occupational therapy shops there is usually available a large size loom with a foot-shifting shed. This gives coördination of hands and feet, flexion and extension of the hips and knees, pulling up and pushing down of the foot, flexion and extension of the shoulders, elbow, wrist, fingers, rotation of the forearm, abduction and adduction of the shoulder, and provides useful, purposeful, coördinated movements of both hands and feet.

Basketry is a valuable craft for spastic children, but it is confined mostly to occupational therapy departments, as it requires the instruction of one trained in this field. It gives valuable exercise, as it requires wide sweeping motions with one hand while the other hand holds the basket in place. It gives abduction of arm, flexion and extension of the fingers, wrist, and elbow.

The work done in occupational therapy departments has the advantage of appealing to the play instinct of the child and carries with it the pleasure of achievement and the reward of praise for work well done.

Vocal Training.—Vocal training is an all-important factor in helping the child, as speech defects are likely to develop personality peculiarities, and cause the child to become introverted. Speech defects also isolate the child from the society of others and accordingly greatly retard his progress. Those trained in speech work can cite many cases of marked improvement in school work, and an increase in the intelligence rating from 10 to 30 per cent after the correction of speech defects. Through it, dull normal persons have become normal, and potential morons have become dull normal persons after vocal training.

If the defect is very severe it may be improved through surgery first, followed by speech training so that the energy expended in uncontrollable motion may be used in better articulation. Speech training will show better results if undertaken after the child has attained some degree of control over his body and has made some progress in coördinating his extremities. Some improvement in speech often follows after the child has had beneficial effects through training in other departments. The training of speech in a spastic child should be undertaken only by one especially equipped and proficient in this science. It is a very slow process and requires patience and persistence, as well as great skill. The individual undertaking speech training should have special training in normal speech mechanisms.

As the muscles of the throat are involved the same as the other muscles of the body, they should have special relaxing exercises. When the child is either lying or sitting comfortably relaxed, gentle massage by superficial stroking of the neck, shoulder, and face muscles is beneficial.

Following massage, the child should take normal and deep breathing exercises. Placing the fingers on the child's tongue steadies and helps relax it. The patient starts with breathing the consonants as p—puh—, etc., and follows with the vowels. He tries to pronounce them on the tip end of the tongue, the tongue and throat drawing up long enough to say the vowel, then relaxing. He takes the vowels one at a time. Later the vowels may be given in sequence, possibly to a tune.

Exercises for the tongue are also good. Pushing the tongue out to a point, spreading it, and bringing it back to a point is the simplest exercise. In another touching first one corner of the mouth then the other, now the upper teeth, then the lower with the end of the tongue, and finally moving the tongue around in a circle appears to the child more fun than exercise.

These exercises may be evolved into a game, thus intriguing the child's interest and coöperation. For the first words, try those resembling natural sounds made by animals such as: moo, baa, etc.

Show the child a picture and call the name of the objects in it. Next give the child short rhymes to learn.

From here progress can be made by having the child compose short sentences to express a thought or a suggested idea.

Teaching the child to sing or whistle affords very good throat exercises.

Having the child practice his word sounding before a mirror is often very beneficial. The child must not be allowed to read aloud until such a time as he is able to enunciate in an understandable manner.

The Spastic as a Unit of Society.— *Relationship of Parents to Child.*— Parents finding themselves faced with the responsibility of rearing a spastic child must resign themselves to this difficult task by adjusting their lives to that of the child. If they work hard to meet the situation with patience and calmness, they will derive more happiness than by endeavoring to find an easy escape. Squarely facing the problem with fortitude and eluding false hopes, they will be able to render the valuable aid of which the child is so sorely in need. The parents should guard against overindulgence of the child, and while exercising a helpful attitude should try to establish a spirit of independence in him. This they can do by encouraging the child to new ventures, at the same time allaying his fears. It is very difficult for the spastic to orient himself to his environment. The problem of acquiring poise and confidence is very similar to that of another individual in overcoming stage fright.

In order to avoid much unhappiness and false steps the parents should discredit all advice from incompetent persons and seek the guidance of a capable orthopedic surgeon.

In order to develop within the child his desire to be part of the "scheme of things," it is well to place him in a group of handicapped children with the same intelligence level. Here he can meet other individuals on an equal footing and can learn to compete, thereby developing a feeling of personal worth. The parents should try to direct into other channels the child's overflow of accumulated energy which interferes with his muscular control. If it is not possible to place him in a good school the parents may arrange to have him study and play with a group of similarly handicapped children. In this way the spastic child will lack the time to sit and watch the activities of normal children, which would tend to make him morbidly introverted and a day dreamer.

If it is possible place the child in a school, for here he will make the necessary adjustments which will enable him to fit more satisfactorily into adult life. Here mental and physical development will progress together along with others like himself and he will be spared the effect of unfair competition so devastating to a child's character.

Recreational and Industrial Prospects.—In the honest endeavor to bring the spastic child to the highest possible mental and physical degree of normality the fact is sometimes overlooked that he has to live in a world of normal persons in which he must strive to sustain himself. Because of his limitations in self-expression, the means should be supplied whereby he may attain an appreciation of art, drama, music and dancing. This can be accomplished by means of self-governed clubs organized for the purposes of study, art and social activities. Here he can enjoy social contact and give expression to their individual preferences in the field of artistic achievements. The spastic can command much better coördination in doing something he enjoys (as in playing a piano) than in doing a routine act, because the factor of his forgetting himself enters in, and his mind centers about the pleasurable activity instead.

If the child has a fair mentality, with an average or a little less than average I. Q., much can be done with the proper vocational and scholastic training within the mental and physical scope of the individual, to enable him to sustain himself industrially.

What a pity it would be to allow the undeveloped natural ability of many an intelligent spastic to go to waste, when with the proper development he would excel many an average citizen, and certainly those who have neglected to use advantageously the favors which nature and opportunity have afforded. The ultimate object is to give society a useful, honest self-supporting individual.

BIBLIOGRAPHY

We are indebted to the following authors of the Bibliography, from whom we have garnered part of our material, and whom we dedicate to the intellectual curiosity of those students who desire to enlarge their knowledge of this subject:

Best, C. H., and Taylor, N. B.: The Living Body, New York, Henry Holt & Company, 1944.

Bowen, W. P.: Applied Anatomy and Kinesiology, 5th ed., Philadelphia, Lea & Febiger, 1934.

Drew, Lillian Curtis: Individual Gymnastics, Edited by Hazel L. Kinzly, 5th ed., Philadelphia, Lea & Febiger, 1945.

EMERSON, C. P., AND TAYLOR, J. E.: Essentials of Medicine, 14th ed., Philadelphia, J. B. Lippincott Company, 1940.

FULTON, J. F.: Muscular Contraction and Reflex Control of Movement, Baltimore, The Williams & Wilkins Company, 1926.

GAENSLEN, F. J.: Aids in Muscle Training, Jour. Am. Med. Assn., March 23, 1935.

GOLDTHWAIT, J. E., BROWN, L. T., SWAIM, L. T., AND KUHNS, J. G.: Essentials of Body Mechanics in Health and Disease, 4th ed., Philadelphia, J. B. Lippincott Company, 1945.

GRAY'S ANATOMY: Edited by Warren H. Lewis, 24th ed., Philadelphia, Lea & Febiger, 1942.

HAWLEY, GERTRUDE: The Kinesiology of Corrective Exercise, Philadelphia, Lea & Febiger, 1937.

HOWELL, W. H.: Textbook of Physiology, 14th ed., Philadelphia, W. B. Saunders Company, 1940.

HOWLAND, I. S.: The Teaching of Body Mechanics in Elementary and Secondary Schools, New York, A. S. Barnes & Company, 1936.

KOVÁCS, R.: A Manual of Physical Therapy, 3rd ed., Philadelphia, Lea & Febiger, 1944.

KRUSEN, F. H.: Physical Medicine, Philadelphia, W. B. Saunders Company, 1941.

LIPOVETZ, JOHN: Applied Physiology of Exercise, Minneapolis, Burgess Publishing Company, 1938.

LIPPITT, LOUISA C.: A Manual of Corrective Gymnastics, New York, The Macmillan Company, 1923.

LOVETT, R. W., OBER, FRANK, AND BRUESTER, A. H.: Lateral Curvature of the Spine and Round Shoulders, Philadelphia, The Blakiston Company, 1931.

LOWMAN, C. L.: Technique of Underwater Gymnastics, Los Angeles, American Publications Inc., 1937.

MACKENZIE, SIR COLIN: The Action of Muscles, New York, Paul B. Hoeber, Inc., 1930.

MACKENZIE, C. W.: Intellectual Development and the Erect Posture, Melbourne, A. Grant, 1924.

MANKELL, N. K., AND KOENIG, E. C.: Posture and Types of Breathing Exercises, New York Med. Jour., **104**, 935, (Nov. 11), 1916.

MCCURDY, J. H., AND LARSON, L. A.: Physiology of Exercise, 3rd ed., Philadelphia, Lea & Febiger, 1939.

MENNELL, J. B.: Physical Treatment by Movement, Manipulation and Massage, 5th ed., Philadelphia, The Blakiston Company, 1945.

MILLARD, NELLIE D., AND KING, B. G.: Human Anatomy and Physiology, Philadelphia, W. B. Saunders Company, 1945.

MOCK, H. E.: Handbook of Physical Therapy, Chicago, Am. Med. Assn., 1939.

MOCK, H. E., COULTER, J. S., AND PEMBERTON, R.: Principles and Practice of Physical Therapy, Vols. I, II and III, Hagerstown, Maryland, W. F. Prior & Company, 1932.

MORRIS' HUMAN ANATOMY: Edited by J. P. Schaeffer, 10th ed., Philadelphia, The Blakiston Company, 1942.

MORRISON, W. R., AND CHENOWETH, L. B.: Normal and Elementary Physical Diagnosis, 3rd ed., Philadelphia, Lea & Febiger, 1941.

MULLINER, MARY REES: Mechano-Therapy, Philadelphia, Lea & Febiger, 1929.

NISSON, HARTVIG: Practical Massage and Corrective Exercises With Applied Anatomy, Philadelphia, F. A. Davis Company, 1929.

PHELPS, W., AND RIPHUTH, R.: The Diagnosis and Treatment of Postural Defects, George Banta Publishing Company, 1932.

QUIRING, D. P., BOYLE, B. A., BOROUSH, E. L., AND LUFKIN, B: The Extremities, Philadelphia, Lea & Febiger, 1945.

SCOTT, M. G.: Analysis of Human Motion, New York, F. S. Crofts & Company, 1942.

SOBOTTA, J., AND MCMURICH, J. P.: Atlas of Human Anatomy, Vols. I, II and III, New York, G. E. Stechert & Company, 1927.

STEINDLER, A.: Mechanics of Normal and Pathological Locomotion in Man, Springfield, Ill., Charles C Thomas, 1935.

THOMAS, L. C., AND GOLDTHWAIT, J. E.: Body Mechanics and Health, Boston, Houghton Mifflin Company, 1929.

WRIGHT, WILHELMINE, G.: Muscle Function, New York, Paul B. Hoeber, Inc., 1928.

INDEX